AIDS: Activism and Alliances

Social Aspects of AIDS
Series Editor: Peter Aggleton
Institute of Education, University of London

AIDS: Activism and Alliances

Edited by

Peter Aggleton, Peter Davies and
Graham Hart

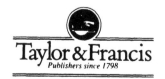

Taylor&Francis
Publishers since 1798

First published 1997
By Taylor & Francis,
11 New Fetter Lane, London EC4P 4EE

Transferred to Digital Printing 2004

A Catalogue Record for this book is available from the British Library

ISBN 0 7484 0575 5
ISBN 0 7484 0576 3 pbk

Library of Congress Cataloging-in-Publication Data are available on request

Series cover design by Barking Dog Art

Typeset in 10/12 pt New Baskerville
by Graphicraft Typesetters Ltd., Hong Kong

Contents

Contents

Preface

Peter Aggleton, Peter Davies and Graham Hart

The eighth conference on the Social Aspects of AIDS took place in London in September 1995, organized around the themes of activism and alliances. As in previous years, it brought together workers in social and behavioural research, community and voluntary groups, health education and health promotion, counselling and care. The choice of themes for the meeting was deliberate, since the time seemed opportune to examine what has been learned about the nature and effects of different kinds of community organizing around AIDS, as well as the different alliances that have come into being as a result of the epidemic. A wide range of papers were presented at the meeting, including many of those contained in this book.

As editors, it has again been a privilege to work with an extraordinarily committed team of people before, during and after the conference. They include Sue Beardsell, Paul Broderick, Carolina Cordero, Andrea Cornwall, Gaby Critchley, Gail Darke, Katherine Donovan, Su Harradine, Brian Heaphy, Laurie Henderson, Ford Hickson, Paul Holland, Peter Keogh, Vijay Kumari, David Reid, Peter Weatherburn and Jeffrey Weeks. Michael Stephens was responsible for overall conference organization. Helen Thomas liaised with contributors in sometimes challenging circumstances, and prepared the manuscript for publication.

Chapter 1

Positive Women and Heterosexuality: Problems of Disclosure of Serostatus to Sexual Partners

June Crawford, Sonia Lawless and Susan Kippax

In Australia, the HIV/AIDS epidemic has been and continues to be one which affects mainly homosexually active men, and one which is concentrated among those who are attached to the central gay communities of Sydney and Melbourne. Since the beginning of the epidemic, 926 women have been diagnosed as HIV antibody positive, and this represents 5 per cent of all HIV positive diagnoses (National Centre in HIV Epidemiology and Clinical Research, 1995).

Australia is frequently cited as one of the success stories in controlling the HIV/AIDS epidemic, and this success is characterized as having been brought about by a 'partnership' model of response to the epidemic. The partnership is that between government, non-governmental organizations and the affected groups and communities. Out of this approach have come models of care and support, prevention and education programmes developed largely by and for gay male communities. Services for women, where they exist at all, have often been grafted on to those for gay men. Women are therefore marginalized within an epidemic which is largely one among gay men. When support services for people living with HIV/AIDS are developed by and for gay male communities, women living with HIV/AIDS are frequently faced with a choice between accessing services which are HIV-friendly but not necessarily woman-friendly and accessing those (such as Women's Health Centres) which are woman-friendly but not necessarily HIV-friendly. In either case, they are made aware of their marginalized status (Lawless, Crawford and Kippax, in press). At the same time, HIV-related services designed to meet the specific needs of women, such as those catering for women with children, women as carers, and women's reproductive needs are largely non-existent (Mkwananzi, 1991).

Disclosure of one's serostatus is a problem for all people living with HIV (Marks *et al.*, 1992; Hays *et al.*, 1993). Research indicates that problems of disclosure, particularly to a sexual partner, constitute a source of stress for HIV-positive people (Hays *et al.*, 1993). For positive women within a largely gay male epidemic, the process of disclosure and fear of breaches of confidentiality are issues of deep concern (O'Sullivan and Thomson, 1992; Simoni *et al.*, 1995).

In New South Wales, where the women who took part in this study lived, the law states that it is an offence for a person who is infected with HIV to engage in sex without informing the sexual partner of their HIV serostatus. This chapter aims to develop an understanding of some of the problems faced by HIV-positive women in disclosing their serostatus to a sexual partner (or potential sexual partner).

Method

The analysis offered here has been informed by data from 27 interviews with women living with HIV. The interviews, which were unstructured, took the form of guided conversations. They were conducted at a location and time nominated by the women, and lasted between three-quarters of an hour and two hours. The topics covered in the interviews included family relationships; sexuality; friendship and support networks; state of health; and experience of health care and HIV-related services. The interviews were tape-recorded and transcribed. In order to ensure confidentiality, all identifying information was removed during transcription. The majority of the women interviewed lived in or were primarily accessing services in the greater Sydney metropolitan area at the time of interview. Further interviews are being conducted in Melbourne. To complement the women's accounts of their experiences, interviews with healthcare workers have also been conducted. This chapter, however, is based only on the women's accounts.

Women were recruited into the study in a number of ways: via the distribution of fliers in doctors' offices, clinics, AIDS Councils and Family Planning Clinics; by referral from various support groups for women living with HIV/AIDS such as Positive Women; by referral from medical and other health professionals; and through snowballing, networking and word of mouth. The women's ages ranged from 22 to 55 years; half of the women were in the 30–35 age range. They were predominantly heterosexual and 45 per cent of the women had either one or two children, almost all of whom were under the age of ten. Sixty-eight per cent of the women were in a sexual relationship at the time of interview and the majority of their partners were HIV antibody negative. Just over half the women were tertiary educated. HIV transmission categories are as follows: 44 per cent heterosexual; 23 per cent medically acquired; 18 per cent injecting drug use (IDU); 15 per cent unknown. This pattern of mode of HIV transmission is very similar to that found in the population of HIV positive women (National Centre in Epidemiology and Clinical Research, 1995).

Analysis

The transcripts of interview were analysed using the principles of grounded theory. Transcripts of the interviews were analysed in terms of similarity and difference (Glaser and Strauss, 1967; Strauss, 1987) and a number of common themes emerged from the accounts of the women. The narratives are not treated as necessarily true accounts but nor are they considered to be false in any sense. Rather, the ways in which the women attempt to make sense of their experience of living with HIV reveal the contradictions and tensions inherent in the prevailing discourses and their positioning within them.

From the outset of this study, it was found that HIV-positive women were very difficult to contact. It became evident that fear of disclosure of their HIV serostatus was the main factor rendering contact difficult. One of the aims of the project as a whole was to develop an understanding of this fear and the social isolation that went with it. In a previous paper, we have shown (Lawless, Crawford and Kippax, in press) how HIV-positive women are positioned by discourses relating to sex, disease and drugs as well as by the dominant discourses surrounding women and HIV/AIDS. We found that women to some extent take on the stigma carried by these dominant discourses.

Discursive Construction of the Positive Woman

Although men living with HIV are also stigmatized (Schaefer and Coleman, 1992; Hays *et al.*, 1993; Hickman *et al.*, 1994), positive gay men in Australia have been exposed to education campaigns which provide alternative discourses and images relating to being a person living with HIV. Shame, guilt and contamination are played down in these discourses, which have sought to promote the sharing of responsibility for transmission among the positive and negative alike.[1]

Gay men acquire HIV by engaging in a practice – anal intercourse – which is one way in which men are identified as gay. Women, on the other hand, when diagnosed as HIV antibody positive, are faced with the need for the reconstruction of self. The discourses available are those associated with deviance, disease and contamination. They can no longer see themselves as 'ordinary' heterosexual women, but find themselves classed as 'promiscuous', deviant and dangerous. They are positioned as a 'polluted source' of infection. In their accounts of their experiences surrounding diagnosis, the women reveal that they are understood by others and also by themselves in terms of these dominant discourses. In the course of interviews conducted here, we found that this is the case regardless of the way in which they became infected with HIV. Whether they acquired HIV medically, through sexual contact or injecting drug use, they expressed the view that they were perceived by others (and hence to some extent perceived themselves) to be stigmatized: dirty, diseased and undeserving (Lawless, Crawford and Kippax, in press). Such stigma functioned as a powerful disincentive to disclosure of their serostatus.

For example, all the women who acquired HIV medically reported being counselled to avoid disclosure at any cost. 'They said to tell people that you've got leukemia or cancer. Don't on any account let anyone know that you have AIDS.' Such advice serves to reinforce women's feelings of shame, guilt and contamination and to confirm their fears of discrimination, even when they consider themselves to be 'innocent victims'. Women who acquired HIV sexually, or who are assumed to have done so, reported experiencing guilt and shame, and feelings of contamination, whether they had had many sexual partners or were infected by a husband or partner within a relationship where they (the women) were monogamous. For example, one woman from the latter group said:

> After the anger process came the awful feeling of dirtiness and I can't – I couldn't get out of the shower. I was scrubbing and scrubbing my teeth and I'd come out of the shower all shampooed and scrubbed and clean and polished and felt dirty and (laugh) I realized I felt my blood was dirty and my whole flesh was dirty so I mean you can't wash that off.

A few of the women were or had been members of stigmatized groups such as lesbians, sex workers or injecting drug users. For them, being HIV antibody positive was an added stigma. It is important to note that all of the women associated being HIV antibody positive with notions of deviance, being a 'threat to society', contaminated and dangerous. This made disclosure so problematic for them.

What was also very clear from the women's accounts was their need to protect those close to them from stigmatization and its harmful consequences. Women's responsibility for others and the fear that those close to them, particularly children, will be subjected to what has been called 'courtesy stigma' (Goffman, 1963) is perhaps the greatest barrier to disclosure and the source of greatest fear associated with disclosure.

> Women seem terribly scared of being identified because . . . it could be a whole family they're identifying for . . . or putting at risk of being you know sort of discriminated against.

Women are expected to be carers and nurturers, to look after the emotional wellbeing of others. Their own needs, which they may sometimes perceive to be best served by disclosing their serostatus, are subordinated.

Disclosure to Sexual Partners

The women interviewed reported that one of the first things they were told at the time of receiving their diagnosis was the legal requirement that they disclose their serostatus to a sexual partner. Disclosure to a sexual partner occurs in two quite different settings. First, we consider disclosing serostatus to a partner with whom there is an existing sexual relationship at the time of diagnosis. There has recently been some public discussion of this in the Australian press. Members of the medical profession want to be given the right to disclose a patient's HIV serostatus to a sexual partner if the patient refuses to do so. At the moment, such a disclosure is in contravention of medical ethics. Many people (including journalists) appear to see this as relatively non-problematic. Members of the gay community, however, have pointed out that such a change in practice may have undesirable consequences.[2] If patients cannot trust their medical practitioner to maintain confidentiality, some may be reluctant to disclose to the medical practitioner, they may be less likely to have an HIV test and thus more likely to transmit HIV. In many ways it seems preferable for medical practitioners (and others) to maintain confidentiality, at the same time providing appropriate counselling to assist the person to disclose to their sexual partner.

Among the women who participated in the study reported here, there were none who failed to disclose their serostatus in an ongoing sexual relationship.[3] This is not to say that there were not problems associated with such disclosure, as the following quote shows:

> because I'd used drugs earlier in my life and I hadn't used them for four years I thought it [the virus] had just come out and I had given it to him. I thought it was all my fault. It was enough to want to start using again. I felt so guilty I couldn't look at him. I thought I had killed someone . . . and then they told me he was bisexual.

For this woman, her diagnosis as HIV-antibody positive brought immediate feelings of guilt, shame and responsibility. Problems associated with disclosure to an existing partner were not about whether or not to disclose, but rather regarding how to come to terms with the enormity of what disclosure might mean. Several women reported being faced with the prospect that they might have been responsible for infecting sexual partners and children. In most cases they were offered little or no help in disclosing this information. The potential for relationships to break down at the very time when the woman may be in most need of the reassurance of continued support from a partner should be recognised by ensuring the provision of appropriate counselling and support services including, but not confined to, peer support.

Only one of the participants in the study reported being offered 'couples' counselling.

We emphasize that the problems associated with disclosure to a sexual partner were evident among all women in existing relationships, including those who were not faced with the necessity to disclose that they had had sex outside of the relationship. Women nevertheless sometimes expressed the view that they felt as if they needed to prove that they had not been 'promiscuous', or injecting drug users. This contributed to the difficulties associated with informing their partner.

It is in relation to new partners that disclosure assumes its most problematic face. In this context, women are faced with several dilemmas. There are a number of ways in which they attempt to resolve these dilemmas, none of which is entirely successful. As described elsewhere (Lawless *et al.*, 1996) some of the women reported that they had avoided such problems by choosing to remain celibate or by choosing positive partners. One woman reported renewing her relationship with the bisexual man who had infected her because it was just too difficult to contemplate seeking a relationship with someone else.

In analysing accounts from women who were faced with a situation in which decisions about disclosure to new sexual partners had to be made, we found that a number of competing and contradictory discourses underpinned their understandings of their experience. As one example, the safe sex[4] discourse which positions all women, and HIV-positive women in particular, as responsible for protecting sexual partners by ensuring consistent condom use (Lawless *et al.*, 1996) is somewhat at odds with the discourse which imposes a legal requirement on those living with HIV to inform potential sexual partners of their serostatus. For if the safe-sex discourse can be relied on, there should be no need to inform a sexual partner of seropositivity.

Heterosexual sexual encounters are to some extent problematic for women generally and, as shown elsewhere (Kippax *et al.*, 1990; Holland, Ramazanoglu and Scott, 1992; Crawford, Kippax and Waldby, 1994) discourses which construct meanings surrounding such encounters are somewhat incompatible with the safe-sex discourse. As shown in the examples discussed in detail below, discourses which construct heterosexuality with particular reference to responsibility, commitment and intimacy (Kippax *et al.*, 1990) are implicated in women's understandings and experiences of heterosexual encounters. These discourses are often conflicting and contradictory.

Hollway (1984) identified three dominant discourses of heterosexuality that frame many heterosexual encounters and relationships. The first of these was identified as the 'strong male sex drive' discourse which positions men as to some extent at the mercy of their hormones, as part of 'nature'. According to this discourse, women are passive, compliant, always ready to satisfy men's needs. One of the contradictions inherent in this discourse is that they also have a duty to 'save themselves' for the 'fittest' male. Women's duty to remain 'pure' requires them to control the uncontrollable. Although denied an active desire of their own, women are deemed to be responsible for what happens in a sexual encounter.

It has been argued elsewhere (Kippax *et al.*, 1990) that the two remaining discourses identified by Hollway are variants of the male sex-drive discourse. The 'to-have-and-to-hold' discourse is that of coupledom, the committed relationship. It is inherent in the marriage contract, allowing the male partner to satisfy his strong sex drive by providing him with unlimited access to one woman's body (Pateman, 1988). The 'to-have-and-to-hold' discourse is based on mutual trust and fidelity.

The third discourse is labelled the 'permissive' discourse, whereby women and men have equal entitlement to 'casual' sex. It is in the context of the 'one-night stand', where emotional involvement and intimacy are not required, that heterosexual relationships may be understood in terms of the permissive discourse. Honesty and trust occupy a problematic position in this discourse; although in theory there should be no reason for either partner to be other than open and honest, it is not unusual for coercion, misunderstandings, deception and misplaced trust to occur (Gavey, 1992).

These three discourses, particularly understandings framed around the construct of the 'strong male sex drive', position women as virgin, wife/mother or 'whore'. Within these discourses, a woman living with HIV/AIDS is an anomaly. She cannot occupy the position of virgin or wife/mother and the position of 'whore' is problematic. As someone who is polluted, the 'carrier' of a life-threatening disease, she is unworthy to be a sex object.

The discourses through which heterosexual encounters are understood are not coherent, nor are they mutually exclusive. A particular encounter is rarely unambiguously one thing or another, a one-night stand or the beginning of a beautiful romance. Discourses themselves are fluid and subject to constant renegotiation and transformation, as new (or even familiar) contradictions arise.

In their attempts to deal with heterosexual encounters with new or potential sex partners, women who are HIV seropositive must deal with the contradictions posed by these conflicting discourses. Heterosexual encounters to some extent are no longer familiar territory. HIV-positive women are faced with the necessity to renegotiate and transform some of the meanings of heterosexual encounters and cannot rely on the other participant in the encounter (that is, the heterosexual man involved) to share their understandings. The following two accounts – one of an encounter in which the woman discloses her serostatus and the other an account of what happens to a woman who decides not to disclose – are striking examples incorporating many of the themes which emerged from the study. Apart from illustrating the potency of the dominant discourses just described, overlaid with the safe-sex discourse, particular themes that emerged include the fear of rejection and violence, responsibility, intimacy and trust. The discussion that follows the excerpts points to the way in which these accounts exemplify some of the contradictions among these constructs and the women's attempts to resolve them.

Marilyn

I had to tell somebody that I was HIV positive and I'd never had to do that before and it was fucking hideous. It's the worst thing I've ever had to do in my life, you know, somebody that is absolutely drop-dead gorgeous and you think well if I told them they might reject me. I think nobody likes rejection you know and with something that's as intimate as that and . . . and it is horrific . . . first of all he said 'Oh, well, that's all right' – he was quite nice actually initially and sort of got a bit watery-eyed and said 'Oh, who's going to look after you' . . . and said 'Oh, he was prepared to have protected sex with me' but then the condom broke and I got my period 'cause I haven't had penetration for over a year and so [it] came early, I mean it was the worst scenario you could possibly imagine and· he bailed me up in a corner for two hours and accused me of being a murdering bitch and I should be locked away and I shouldn't be allowed to be attractive and . . . you know it was hideous. I didn't know if I was going to walk out of there alive.

Sarah

I know even in NSW it's the law to tell them before you enter into – ah – I'm sorry I didn't. I broke the law . . . (laugh). Um, I did ensure that we had protected sex and there was – I talked to him about personal responsibility and I – he didn't want to wear condoms and he didn't, he said 'Well, you know, I'm clean and you're clean'. I was like look I'm fastidious but you don't know what I've got. It's not about what someone else's got, I tried to explain to him, it was about what he was prepared to expose himself to and as he had no idea of who I was really, and I had no idea who he was, it was nothing to do with that. It was about what I was prepared to expose myself to and felt safe with as an individual. So I tried to educate him while I was doing that [be]cause it was something he had no concept of at all (sigh) . . . in 1995. Umm . . . he had an understanding that AIDS was around, umm . . . and people get HIV but it was pretty limited stuff. So anyway it took me a month to tell him and then I did it when we were both in bed with no clothes on and it was like I've got something to tell you [laugh] and he jumped out of bed and he put his clothes on very quickly and ran up and down the corridor saying he didn't know what to do. He said really vile things too but it was very bizarre. He actually moved into my house the same day and then wouldn't talk to me for three days and that was horrible.

It really hurt, yeah, and it's that thing of . . . like you've tricked me, you've sucked me in and now you're letting me know and it was like so I was meant to tell you when I first met you? I still would have been your friend. I said I've more . . . friends than I know what to do with. I want a lover, I want a mate, I want somebody that I can be particularly intimate with . . . and it was like he just had to accept it and that everything would be okay and run smoothly.

These are two different attempts to solve the same problem. Marilyn's encounter may have been successful if the condom had not broken, but nevertheless this account reveals a potential for violence whenever something goes wrong. She had tried to do the right thing: she informed her male partner of her status and he 'said he was prepared to' engage in protected sex with her in full knowledge of the circumstances. Nevertheless, when the condom broke (and it is not clear whether he carried any responsibility for the breakage) he is described as taking no responsibility for what happened. He is described as becoming verbally violent and is also judged by the woman to be potentially physically violent ('I didn't know if I was going to walk out of there alive').

This account points to the strangeness and unfamiliarity of the situation ('I'd never had to do that before and it was fucking hideous'). Marilyn's account links intimacy with disclosing her serostatus ('something that's as intimate as that'). Intimacy is incompatible with the 'permissive' discourse which generally applies to understandings surrounding the 'one-night stand'. The account of the man's reaction when the condom broke invokes the 'male sex drive' discourse – women are 'too attractive', seductive and irresponsible. On the other hand, women are held responsible for whatever happens in the sexual encounter.

In the case of Sarah, she did not disclose her serostatus until after a sexual relationship had been formed. Disclosing under these circumstances also brought a very real possibility of rejection. Her partner's reaction was in some respects even more judgemental than that of the man in Marilyn's account. In both cases, the man's reaction was in terms of accusation directed at the woman. She is characterized as a vile seductress, with no right to be 'so attractive'. A positive woman is deemed to have no right to a sex life, and her positive status appears to be a real threat to men's confidence in their ability to differentiate between 'clean' and 'unclean' women (Waldby, Kippax and Crawford, 1993).

These and other accounts point to the contradictions faced by positive women in their efforts to engage in any sort of sex life. The meanings attached to heterosexual relations are informed by the dominant discourses surrounding heterosexuality (Hollway, 1984), including the strong male sex drive discourse (particularly evident in Marilyn's account above) and the to-have-and-to-hold discourse implicated in Sarah's account.

As pointed out, women find disclosure of serostatus extremely problematic. They often do not disclose even to close family members and friends.

How can disclosing to a (new) sexual partner fail to be a source of extreme concern? As shown in Sarah's account, some women go to a great deal of trouble to ensure that it is 'safe' to disclose their serostatus. The discourse of responsibility is invoked in her account of how she prepared for disclosure. In common with the accounts of many other women, she stresses her role as 'educator' of her partner and points to the need to educate him in general terms even before he agrees to have protected sex.

In order to disclose her serostatus, Sarah needs to have achieved the greatest possible degree of intimacy with her partner. She chooses a moment when they are both in bed naked together. She finally feels safe to disclose, and in her account it appears that this is an act designed to increase intimacy, to strip away one more barrier, in order to get nearer to her partner. There are conflicting and contradictory discourses operating here. On the one hand, Sarah knows that she risks rejection by disclosing her serostatus. But the more important the relationship is to her, the more important it is not to maintain secrecy from him. Trust is central to discourses of coupledom (Stephenson, 1994). Disclosing her serostatus also means disclosing implicit dishonesty, so that in being honest she is confessing to having been dishonest. Her disclosure reveals not only that she is seropositive, but also that she is not to be trusted.

Moral dilemmas and paradoxes of this kind are faced by any woman who has 'something to hide' when entering into a sexual relationship. In the case of HIV seropositivity, however, what has been 'hidden' is especially loaded. The revelation of a woman's 'secret' threatens her partner on multiple levels. It threatens his view of himself as someone who is capable of selecting 'clean' partners. It makes him feel that he too is contaminated. It also poses a real threat that he has in fact been infected (although it should not do so if the couple had practised only protected intercourse).

As noted by Wilton and Aggleton (1991, p. 155): 'Women who attempt to negotiate safer sex with male partners risk abuse, physical violence or the loss of that partner, often with profound social and economic consequences.' As in Sarah's account above, the accounts of positive heterosexual women are similar to those of other heterosexual women when it comes to persuading a man to use condoms. The placing of the responsibility for safe sex on to women (whether HIV-positive or not) is another instance of conflicting discourses. For those women who are not living with HIV, they have a choice between insisting on condom use and risking becoming infected. Their discursive positioning as passive and self-sacrificing disallows insistence if there is any resistance on the part of a man to the use of the condom, and they consent to unprotected sex 'for his sake'. Such a course of action is not available to a woman who is HIV seropositive. If she permits unprotected sexual intercourse, she is putting him at risk. She thus has a stronger commitment to safe sex and in some cases may disclose her serostatus in order to ensure that he himself is not put at risk.

Although the positive women's accounts did not include accounts where disclosure took place because of the man's refusal to use a condom, Sarah's account of her first sexual encounter with her partner suggests that she came close to doing so. Another woman described an encounter in which she persuaded her partner to use a condom; he then suggested that now that he had done it 'her way' he was entitled to do it 'his way' (that is, without a condom).

> He said 'Yeah, yeah, that's fine' and I thought 'Great, you know, I'm getting really good at negotiating this stuff,' took him home and we had sex once and that was fine but then it was his turn . . . and it was like 'Okay, well, I've worn the condom for you but now like it's your turn to let me enjoy it' . . . which meant him not wearing a condom the second time around. I thought no way, so I like had this man sitting naked at the end of my bed saying 'But I haven't got anything' and I didn't kind of feel it was appropriate to disclose at that point . . . I just like said 'Well, forget it, then' and sent him home.

Conclusions

Women's problems of disclosure of their serostatus to sexual partners are highlighted by the above analysis. It is likely that similar problems are experienced by gay men and by other HIV-seropositive persons. Comparable research on other groups is obviously needed. We argue, however, that, in the Australian context, where the great majority of people living with HIV are gay men, disclosure is particularly problematic for women.

The association of the HIV epidemic in Australia with homosexually active men means that women (and heterosexual men) are automatically assumed to be HIV negative, as illustrated by the above accounts from women. For most women, their construction of self is that of someone who is 'normal', mainstream and unremarkable. For such women, the process of disclosure is one with which they may be totally unfamiliar; stigma itself is likely to be an entirely new experience. Unlike gay men, who have almost certainly known someone who is HIV positive (Prestage *et al.*, 1995), the women interviewed had very limited contact with the HIV epidemic before becoming HIV positive. They thus have no role models of disclosure on which to draw.

A major component of the problematic nature of disclosure of serostatus for HIV-positive women relates to discourses which position positive women as dirty, diseased and undeserving (Lawless, Crawford and Kippax, in press). This is not necessarily the case with respect to HIV-positive gay men. The activity which brings about HIV infection for a gay man is one that is not stigmatized within gay male communities. It is widely practised (Prestage *et al.*, 1995) and, although seen as a 'perversion' by mainstream society, is 'normal' and 'natural' for many gay men. Although the 'act' by which women become infected is most frequently heterosexual intercourse, the discourses surrounding positive women do not position them as 'normal'. They are judged to have engaged in sex in some context which is deviant: too frequently or with the wrong person or in the 'wrong' way. A woman who becomes HIV-positive has to re-evaluate her whole sense of self.

Positive women's accounts confirm that self-disclosure of their serostatus to others can be done only with great difficulty. In the case of disclosure to sexual partners, particularly new or potential sexual partners, the situation for positive women is complex and contradictory. Seropositivity is like an invisible stigma. Unless some action is taken, it is unlikely to be revealed. This places responsibility on the positive woman to make decisions about disclosure.

In a heterosexual relationship, disclosure may involve the possibility not only of rejection but also of verbal or physical violence. Although not mentioned by any of the women, disclosure may also pose the risk that the person who has been told will himself disclose the woman's serostatus to others, possibly to people that the woman would wish to remain unaware of her serostatus. In a sexual relationship that is more than 'casual', one that is ongoing and meaningful in the woman's life, there is the added risk that disclosure will mean the end of a relationship which may be very important for her.

The discursive positioning of women as caring, nurturing and responsible when interacting with that of seropositivity, which positions a positive woman as dirty, diseased and irresponsible, renders the disclosure of serostatus exceptionally problematic. Despite the problems on which this chapter has focused, many of the positive women interviewed reported that they eventually found ways of forming new relationships. Their accounts reveal that, for the most part, they are resourceful and persevering, getting on with their lives.

One of the ways in which positive women's lives can be made easier is to challenge the dominant discourse surrounding the 'positive woman'. What is needed is a recognition that women who are HIV-positive are likely to have become infected through heterosexual intercourse, often within a committed relationship such as marriage. For them, as for gay men, the act which brought about their seropositive status is not perverted or unnatural. A discursive reconstruction of the 'positive woman' also needs to recognize that women living with HIV have the right to a sex life, the right to a sexual relationship and the right to be respected. Simplistic messages to 'always have safe sex' and that it is a positive person's legal duty to inform potential sexual partners of their seropositivity are likely to be counterproductive.

Acknowledgments

We should like to express our appreciation to the positive women and their service providers for their participation in this study.

Notes

1 See, for example, posters promoting positive safe sex, including those by Dunbar and McDiarmid and discussion of them by Gott (1994, pp. 202–3).
2 *Sydney Morning Herald*, January 1996. Articles and correspondence about changes to the code of ethics of the Australian Medical Association in order to permit members of the medical profession to breach confidentiality when a person's medical condition and behaviour places others at risk.
3 It is acknowledged that a woman who had not disclosed to her current sexual partner would be very unlikely to have taken part in this study. Many of the women, however, gave information about disclosure in both present and past relationships.
4 We use the term 'safe sex' rather than 'safer sex' since this is the usage in the Australian HIV prevention and education context.

References

CRAWFORD, J., KIPPAX, S. and WALDBY, C. (1994) 'Women's sex talk and men's sex talk', *Feminism and Psychology*, **4**, 4, pp. 571–87.

GAVEY, N. (1992) 'Technologies and effects of heterosexual coercion', in C. KITZINGER, S. WILKINSON and R. PERKINS (Eds) *Special Issue on Heterosexuality, Feminism and Psychology* 2, 3, pp. 325–51.

GLASER, B. and STRAUSS, A. (1967) *The Discovery of Grounded Theory: Strategies for Qualitative Research*, Chicago: Aldine.

GOFFMAN, E. (1963) *Stigma: Notes on the Management of Spoiled Identity*, Englewood Cliffs, NJ: Prentice Hall.

GOTT, T. (1994) 'Where the streets have new aims: The poster in the age of AIDS', in T. GOTT (Ed.) *Don't Leave Me this Way: Art in the Age of AIDS*, Canberra: National Gallery of Australia.

HAYS, R.B., MCKUSICK, L., PALLACK, L., HILLIARD, R., HOFF, C. and COATES, T.L. (1993) 'Disclosing HIV seropositivity to significant others', *AIDS*, **7**, pp. 425–31.

HICKMAN, B., CANNOLD, L., O'LOUGHLIN, B., WOOLCOCK, G., MCLEAN, S. and RAPHAEL, B. (1994) 'Personal relationships and HIV/AIDS', *Venereology*, **7**, 4, pp. 175–81.

HOLLAND, J., RAMAZANOGLU, C. and SCOTT, S. (1992) 'Pleasure, pressure and power: some contradictions of gendered sexuality', *Sociological Review*, **40**, 4, pp. 645–74.

HOLLWAY, W. (1984) 'Women's power in heterosexual sex', *Womens Studies International Forum*, **25**, 1, pp. 63–8.

KIPPAX, S., CRAWFORD, J., WALDBY, C. and BENTON, P. (1990) 'Women negotiating heterosex', *Womens Studies International Forum*, **13**, 6, pp. 533–42.

LAWLESS, S., CRAWFORD, J. and KIPPAX, S. 'Dirty, diseased and undeserving: the positioning of HIV positive women', *Social Science and Medicine* (in press).

LAWLESS, S., CRAWFORD, J., KIPPAX, S. and SPONBERG, M. (1996) '"If it's not on . . .": Heterosexuality for HIV positive women', *Venereology*, **9**, 1, pp. 15–23.

MARKS, G., BUNDEK, N.I., RICHARDSON, J.L., RUIZ, M.S. MALDONADO, M. and MASON, H.R. (1992) 'Self-disclosure of HIV infection to sexual partners', *American Journal of Public Health*, **81**, pp. 1321–2.

MKWANANZI, M. (1991) 'National needs assessment of HIV positive women – Phase I resource package', Sydney, Australia: Macquarie University, NSW.

NATIONAL CENTRE IN HIV EPIDEMIOLOGY AND CLINICAL RESEARCH (1995) *Surveillance Report*, October, **11**, 4.

O'SULLIVAN, S. and THOMSON, K. (Eds) (1992) *Positively Women: Living with AIDS*, London: Sheba Feminist Press.

PATEMAN, C. (1988) *The Sexual Contract*, Cambridge: Polity Press.

PRESTAGE, G., KIPPAX, S., CRAWFORD, J., NOBLE, J., BAXTER, D. and COOPER, D. (1995) 'Method and sample in a study of homosexually active men in Sydney, Australia', Macquarie University: Paper presented at the HIV AIDS and Society Conference, Macquarie University, July.

SCHAEFER, S. and COLEMAN, E. (1992) 'Shifts in meaning, purpose, and values following a diagnosis of human immunodeficiency virus (HIV) infection among gay men', *Journal of Psychology and Human Sexuality*, **1**, pp. 13–29.

SIMONI, J.M., MASON, H.R.C., MARKS, G., RUIZ, M., REED, D. and RICHARDSON, J.L. (1995) 'Women's self-disclosure of HIV infection: rates, reasons and reactions', *Journal of Consulting and Clinical Psychology*, **63**, 3, pp. 474–8.

STEPHENSON, N. (1994) ' "Being true" and telling the truth. The configuration of trust in the talk of young heterosexuals', Paper presented at HIV AIDS and Society Conference, Macquarie University, July.

STRAUSS, A. (1987) *Qualitative Analysis for Social Scientists*, Cambridge: Cambridge University Press.

WALDBY, C., KIPPAX, S. and CRAWFORD, J. (1993) 'Cordon sanitaire: "clean" and "unclean" women in the AIDS discourse of young heterosexual men', in P. AGGLETON, P. DAVIES and G. HART (Eds) *AIDS: Facing the Second Decade*, London: Taylor & Francis.

WILTON, T. and AGGLETON, P. (1991) 'Condoms, coercion and control: heterosexuality and the limits to HIV/AIDS education', in P. AGGLETON, G. HART and P. DAVIES (Eds) *AIDS: Responses, Interventions and Care*, London: The Falmer Press.

Chapter 2

Suffering in Silence? Public Visibility, Private Secrets and the Social Construction of AIDS

Neil Small

In 1986 Roy Cohn died in a US Hospital. He had AIDS, he was a secret homosexual. He was also violently right-wing, a close aid of Joseph McCarthy during the witch hunts and a prosecutor of the Rosenbergs. He is remembered in a panel in the AIDS Memorial Quilt that reads 'Roy Cohn – Coward/Bully/Victim' and he is also remembered in Tony Kushner's *Angels in America* plays. Kushner explores, as one theme in his plays, the question of how broad and embracing the gay sense of community is. Does it encompass an implacable foe like Roy Cohn? At one point Belize, the black gay male nurse caring for Roy, tells him of the likely treatments he will be offered in hospital: radiation and double-blind drug-trial protocols. He advises that these are offered in the interests of medicine and not of the patient and tells Roy to reject them. Roy wants to know why the nurse is telling him this: 'I think you have little reason to want to help me.' Belize replies, 'Consider it solidarity. One faggot to another' (Kushner, 1994, p. 13).

Belize's solidarity here is one born of opposition as well as of humanity. There are other solidarities. Some are born out of positive assertion. Both Cindy Patton and Simon Watney have argued for the importance of using gay pride and gay community values to shape effective HIV prevention (e.g. Watney, 1994). But both have also recognized that there are problems in seeking alliances. Watney reviews European reactions in which governments of the left and of the right have exhibited anti-gay prejudice. Patton (1990) looks to the work of Judith Butler (1990) to consider the problems of coalition politics when they collide with identity politics.

In this chapter I explore the interface between solidarity and identity in relation to HIV and AIDS. In so doing I develop three themes. First, I consider further what identity and solidarity might mean. In particular, I ask if the first can exist in any fixed sense and if the second is desirable if it is predicated on the necessity of alliances. Second, I consider two examples of activity: volunteerism particularly as exemplified in the US via the group Gay Men's Health Crisis, and campaigns to promote and sustain safer sex. Third, I report what a small group of people living with AIDS told me about their thoughts on the private secret of their diagnosis and on identity and solidarity.[1] The argument, therefore, moves from the theoretical, via examples of practice, to the personal.

Identity, Solidarity and the Problems of Alliances

We are not one thing only. We sit at the intersection of different identities. I described Belize above as a 'black gay male nurse' and in so doing incorporated into one throwaway phrase something about his race, sexuality, gender and social status. We cannot assume that these identities sit easily together. Patton argues that although persons situated at the junctures of multiple identities and issue points should not have to choose their allegiances, in effect 'the tendency to totalisation in coalition efforts practically boils down to just such painful choices' (Patton, 1990, p. 163). Butler (1990) suggests that coalition, or even agreement, may not be a desirable goal, only a strategic or tactical moment. As Foucault (1981) has argued, juridical systems of power produce the subjects they subsequently come to represent. 'The task is to formulate within this constituted frame a critique of the categories of identity that contemporary juridical structures engender, naturalise, and immobilize' (Butler, 1990, p. 5).

The problem here is both one of theory and practice. It is also a problem at the core of contemporary politics. Peter Tatchell, a member of the lesbian and gay human rights group 'OutRage' (he is also many other things, a white gay man, a poet, a writer, an activist in many areas)[2] argues against attempts to assimilate gays and lesbians into 'straight' society. He does not want to give up alliances: these can be used, for example, to fight for law reform. But

> The key to queer advancement is self-help and community empowerment. That way we are less at the mercy of institutions dominated by heterosexuals and more in control of our own destiny. With self-reliance, we can create our own homo-affirming community and safe queer space where we do not have to justify ourselves or plead with heterosexuals for acceptance. We can give each other the support that straight society denies us. (*Observer*, 19 June 1994)

The same sort of argument has been presented by women, by Black people, by the disabled. The problem is: what happens when such identities intersect? Where does a disabled Black lesbian choose to locate herself when her coalition politics collide with her identity politics? Albert Innaurato (1994) uses fiction to probe even deeper when he creates the scenario of two ignoble 'fatties' being jostled and moved along by the beautiful bodies on a gay parade. In so doing he pours scorn on easy notions of community arising automatically from identity politics.

Some of the identities we have looked at are also communicated through, and felt as, stigma. It is not that stigma exists alongside or around a core identity but rather that stigma is the identity, or the subjectivity of the person (see Fox, 1993). The reactions to this situation are varied. Some people confront stigma. There are a number of examples within sexual politics of gay groups seeking to confront and reverse overt and covert discrimination, OutRage and the Stonewall Group are examples in the UK. They serve as activist and lobbying groups but also as 'movements of affirmation' (Watney, 1994, p. 246). In the USA, groups have been set up to combat anti-gay violence: 'Community United Against Violence' in San Francisco and 'Queer Nation', set up in New York in 1990, are examples here (Kayal, 1993). The latter also exhibits another characteristic of affirmation: the wish to subvert, via incorporation, derogatory language.

AIDS, for some, adds further urgency and intensity to the need for affirmation. For others it is a problem to be overcome, or a reason to avoid the public arena. There is now considerable autobiography from people living with AIDS (Small, 1993a). Much of this considers the interaction of stigmas. Emmanuel Dreuilhe asks:

> How can homosexuals and drug addicts feel patriotically inspired in their private war when they don't even like themselves, or may actually hate themselves because of a self-image that reflects society's contempt for them? If the opinion of others finally convinces you that you are morally and physically deficient, how can you believe in yourself or in the importance of survival? (Dreuilhe, 1987, p. 34)

Richie McMullen writes that when he was told he had HIV disease he felt, as an initial response, dirty, guilty and ashamed. Despite, he says, having been 'out' for many years, the pain was in part a shame at being found out. 'My HIV disease had, at that time, the perfect host in which to do its worst. Where had all my development gone?' (McMullen, 1988, p. 24). John Money also contributes to the same point: 'How are you supposed to feel about yourself when you are derided, arrested and called immoral?' (Money, 1987, p. 53).

But there is also affirmation. Money says that nursing a grudge is life-threatening to an ill person and that there is a need to forgive historical trespass. McMullen reminds us that moral projections (we can substitute stigma) say more about the persons who make them than those they are directed at. He concludes: 'I am proud to be associated with an international Gay community which has achieved so much in the field of caring responsibility' (McMullen, 1988, p. 66).

Public visibility and private secrets exist as rationales for responding to

17

stigma. They are not opposites. Rather they sit alongside each other. They are manifestations of subjectivity developed within a scenario that combines ontological insecurity, generated when confronting one's mortality, and social insecurity, when one is surrounded by hostility.

A dilemma for many people is that when they have to live with AIDS as well as with another stigma, they have to confront the extent to which the identity of having AIDS replaces other identities. Paul Monette writes that his diagnosis generated a 'sense of separateness (that) would grow so acute that I really didn't want to talk to anyone any more who wasn't touched by AIDS, body and soul' (Monette, 1988, p. 94).

Will affiliation be possible with other people with AIDS who don't share 'secondary characteristics'? Or will the identity of being someone HIV-positive or someone with AIDS be accommodated as a subset of another identity – being gay, for example? Evidence still needs to be assembled. Attempts to develop care regimes for people with AIDS have experienced problems in 'mixing' gay men and those who acquired HIV infection through shared injecting (see Small, 1993b). In contrast, and undermining the fictional scenario offered by Innaurato above, on 18 June 1994 a march in London to celebrate 25 years of Gay Pride saw a group of disabled people leading the march in their wheelchairs.

We return to Butler's (1990) argument that coalition in identity politics should only be tactical. Anything else risks compromising the very *raison d'être* of the affirmative aspects of identity politics. This is a debate about how far one should aim for affirmation or affiliation and if the latter inevitably undermines the former.

Affirmation and Affiliation in Action

Simon Watney has argued that: 'Gayness . . . provides both an individual and a collective identity, quite unlike the more individualistic term "homosexual", or for that matter "heterosexual". It was without doubt the tenacity of British gay culture in all its myriad forms, that has provided our best defence against HIV' (Watney, 1994, p. 247). Here, I explore aspects of this defence. I also consider Gay Mens Health Crisis as an example of a response to a need by those who appeared most at risk. Philip Kayal believes that it is through the detail of care that has evolved as a response to AIDS that this epidemic 'takes us beyond our everyday assumptions about what illness means, what voluntary work should consist of, and what being political entails. It forcibly brings to light why AIDS has greater sociological significance than its medical and biological dimensions alone suggest' (Kayal, 1993, p. xv).

Both Watney's and Kayal's claims incorporate assumptions about identity and about affirmation. They also suggest that the benefits that come about from those concerned with identity politics can be transmitted to other groups. Cindy Patton argues that those veterans of HIV organizing, and of shifting from research to practice, are 'the policy and prevention experts who should be placed in charge in the next decade of the epidemic' (Patton, cited in King, 1993, p. viii). This is not an argument for affiliation but rather for dissemination. I return to the possible implications of seeking to juxtapose lessons learned in one place to another in my conclusions.

That there was a change in gay men's sexual behaviour in the 1980s is clear. The specifics of the change, its permanence, how far it was change in a cohort rather than a population: these are all items of dispute. It is also clear that this change was a result of factors emerging from within the gay community. It was not to do with the arrival of HIV antibody-testing or of government health-education campaigns. Indeed, as the change was occurring we could see, at the same time, a de-gaying of AIDS when government, press and much of the academic community displayed more concern with 'new' sources of transmission and with 'professional' responses to need. This was a move that ignored the (still) majority who were living with HIV and AIDS and sought to shut off those lessons about behaviour change that came from peer experience.[3]

It was the process of peer endorsement of safer sex, informed and reinforced by the gay press and gay groups, that led to behaviour change. This shift was 'founded upon gay men's sense of shared interests and responsibility for each other, and upon individual and collective determination to overcome this latest threat' (King, 1993, pp. 75–6). We see here an example in practice of Watney's sense that 'gay' incorporates, *ipso facto*, community, and of Tatchells' recognition of the benefits of self-help and community empowerment.

Gay Mens Health Crisis (GMHC) began in an *ad hoc* way in New York in 1981. It obtained its corporate charter in 1982 and by the early 1990s had a yearly budget approaching $20 million and an active volunteer corps of over 2000. By the end of 1992 the organization had actively helped nearly 14 000 people with AIDS. 'Until 1988, AIDS, GMHC, and the gay community had been coterminous with each other. They evolved together' (Kayal, 1993, p. 3). The moving forces behind this response were homophobia and volunteerism. 'Gay/AIDS volunteerism was created and given its political character by AIDS-homophobia, wherein gay people and their lives are further denounced because of AIDS and the disease is disavowed because it is thought to be gay' (Kayal, 1993, p. 5).

In recent years there have been changes in GMHC, caused partly by the changing picture of the epidemic and in part to do with the structural dynamics of rapidly developed organizations. Specialist organizations have developed to respond to the needs of women with AIDS and to the needs of members of minority cultures. Among gays a new style of assertion is evident in ACT-UP and in Queer Nation. Volunteers today in GMHC are more inclined to see the work they do there as part of a series of things they are active in, in contrast to 'a whole generation of gay men (for whom) AIDS was the only thing to be concerned about if one wanted to live' (Kayal, 1993, p. 228). Amid this GMHC has been left as a corporate entity with often bureaucratic concerns. We can see the routinization of charisma and the difficulty of avoiding ossification that has been evident in many areas of imaginative and challenging innovation.[4]

In considering safer sex education, and the various activities to care about and care for people with AIDS evident in GMHC, we can see the progress that has been made through affirmation. Peer pressure and volunteerism both link to identity and pride. The benefits of affiliation are more elusive. There are some one-way benefits. The lessons learned by AIDS activists have raised major questions of widespread relevance: about drug policies including testing and the use of placebos, about what confidentiality means in practice, about how the views of service users and carers must be located centrally in a research process that should be reflective, and so on (see Small, 1993a). The benefits of affiliation for gay groups are more difficult to identify. A diminution of identity politics and therefore a shift from the very thing that gave strength to the movement, appears more likely.

Public Visibility and Private Secrets

At the point in *Angels in America* when Roy Cohn is given his diagnosis, he tells his doctor that he does not have AIDS. Poor people and people with no important contacts have AIDS: he has liver cancer. Diagnosis is about social power and not about immune systems. Using social power allows him to avoid stigma, the assumed secondary characteristics he believes will be added to a publically known AIDS diagnosis.

Everyone diagnosed as HIV-positive has to negotiate the extent to which this will remain a secret. Choices and strategies vary considerably. One man, living with his wife and children in the north of England, told me: 'I tell people I have got leukaemia. Then they are with you. So why can't they be with you if you tell them what is really wrong with you?' He continued: 'I think you convince yourself that you have actually got leukaemia. It gets to the situation when there is something about leukaemia on the television, you listen and you think "Well, that's no good." Then it suddenly hits you that you haven't got it.' This strategy keeps stigma at bay, in this man's view. But it does cut off him, and his family, from the support of people also living with AIDS.

Another man living with his family in the same town tells how his diagnosis has:

> affected the family, work, friends, everything. There is not much that
> you can say about it to anybody. It's such a stinker of a thing. Perhaps

if we could talk about it more openly with people it would take the pressure off, it wouldn't be so bad. But you can't really say anything because . . . everybody's tarred with the same brush. I've got what you might call the easy bit. When I go I won't have to live with it any more but everyone else has to. So it doesn't finish with death, does it?

This man also told people he had cancer: 'It's still unexplained but at least it's accepted.'

A man in London, also living with AIDS, offers a different setting but a similar reluctance to tell people his diagnosis. 'By being gay, being single and male you are living with people who know that they may come into contact with the virus anyway. If you tell people too much about it they get uptight.' He had told his mother but not most of his friends. He was worried that if he did, he might drive them away. 'All you do is think of me me me. It's quite unfair sometimes because you neglect other people.' When he did tell friends, one response in particular was surprising. 'He told me, "There's something I've been meaning to tell you. I'm awfully sorry to have to tell you but I'm HIV positive as well".'

Maintaining private secrets is understandable when we relate it to the public profile of the epidemic. It is also understandable as a personal choice, made outside any social determinants. But it has an impact on the capacity to access support for oneself and one's carers and to contribute to, and benefit from, solidarity and affirmation. As the three people quoted above demonstrate, their secrets are not kept from everyone but they draw a line beyond which they will not go.

The role of solidarity, and the reality of community, can have an ambiguous impact on peoples' lives. One man, diagnosed as HIV-positive very early in the epidemic in Britain, told me how he saw his access to some savings and to his own house as being of crucial importance.

It is stress and financial worry and vile surroundings that you can't escape from. There isn't anything wrong with ghettos, there is a lot of warmth. It's when you can't get out that the problems start, which of course is what any disease does, it puts you in a ghetto. Now if you can get out, that's OK when you feel like it, no matter for how long. Just the sheer knowledge that you can get out. But when you have no clout and you are constantly cap in hand, I mean that must drain.

Others struggle: they recognize that identity, community and solidarity do not automatically spring up together. One man had moved to London, attracted by the opportunities to be involved in a gay culture. He had AIDS and spoke about seeing a man in a gay club. 'He had a red face. You could see it was . . . and you get so upset seeing things like that. I think the people who are able to say today, "You don't die with AIDS, you live with it", it's a very positive attitude, but it is very hard to be able to reach that point and I haven't been able to reach it.'

Another man in London, and actively involved in gay life there, described how:

> a couple of my friends, when they have been diagnosed and now they have developed full blown, their friends just shied away from them. That's very hurtful, it grieves me to think . . . I count my blessings. I do have good friends. I know if I were to develop the 'Big A' then they wouldn't shun me. But, you know, for some people that can kill. Because the departure would be so crippling and the stress on the person with the disease would be so unbearable it really does put them back to zero. They don't realize this, you know. If people are so scared about the disease why don't they ask about it?

Private secrets do not stop people benefiting in some areas of their lives from the self-help movements that constitute a part of the public visibility of the epidemic. But when secrets sit alongside fear or denial, then, at the very least, pride and solidarity are absent. One can benefit vicariously but not contribute – and contribution has for many been life-enhancing throughout this epidemic.

Conclusions

I have examined some of the ways that identity and solidarity have been formulated and have considered how far coalition politics and identity politics can coexist in relation to HIV and AIDS. I sought to locate these concerns through the examples of safer sex education and the voluntarism evident in Gay Mens Health Crisis. I continued by considering some examples of people with AIDS talking about their relationship with friends and with the wider world and, specifically, considered the place of secrets.

Out of this material a number of problems emerge. When a person is living with AIDS, what becomes the dominant characteristic that defines, for them, their place in the world? Is it their diagnosis or is it another, pre-existing, characteristic – gender, race or sexuality perhaps? How far can solidarity be generated around an identity of 'person with AIDS' without accompanying secondary characteristics? Will pride and affirmation be inevitably eroded by alliance?

Underpinning many of these questions is a policy dimension. We must ask, first: is a systematic de-gaying of AIDS likely to lead to a loss of the impetus that has done most to generate both prevention and care? Second, how can the benefits of the achievements of gay men be transferred to other groups who do not share the resource of pride and the mechanisms of affirmation? The first is answered easily, yes – but a politics of opposition remains and offers hope. The second is more difficult. We must examine the construction of identity and the nature of solidarity among other groups. We must develop a critique of the nature of stigma and of the impact of secrets. Eventually we need to return to theorizing social power and its impact on the disempowered, and construct strategies for change and for care that encompass the realization that HIV and AIDS are a private concern but also, and not paradoxically, a public issue – an issue of politics.

Notes

1   Between 1989 and 1993 I was involved in research into aspects of living with AIDS. Part of that research involved close contact with a small number of people living with AIDS in London and in a city in the north of England. Our discussions were wide-ranging and included the topics developed in this chapter. I quote those who were enthusiastically supportive of my seeking a wider audience for their thoughts. Their names have been changed.
2   I will now stop listing people's various 'identities' – I hope the point has been made!
3   It is not my intention here to go into detail about these debates. They are well covered, with extensive references, in King (1993).
4   The routinization of charismatic organizations was first observed by Max Weber in relation to religious groups. Latterly it has been discussed in relation to the practice of the therapeutic community (see Manning, 1989) and the hospice movement (see James and Field, 1992).

References

BUTLER, J. (1990) *Gender Trouble*, London: Routledge.

DREUILHE, E. (1987) *Mortal Embrace. Living with AIDS*, London: Faber and Faber.

FOUCAULT, M. (1981) *The History of Sexuality*, Harmondsworth: Penguin Books.

FOX, N. (1993) *Postmodernism, Sociology and Health*, Buckingham: Open University Press.

INNAURATO, A. (1994) 'Solidarity', in G. STAMBOLIAN (Ed.) *Men on Men 2*, Harmondsworth: Plume.

JAMES, N. and FIELD, D. (1992) 'The routinization of hospice: charisma and bureaucratization', *Social Science and Medicine*, **34**, pp. 1363–75.

KAYAL, P.M. (1993) *Bearing Witness*, Oxford: Westview Press.

KING, E. (1993) *Safety in Numbers*, London: Cassell.

KUSHNER, T. (1994) *Angels in America, Part Two: Perestroika*, London: Nick Hern Books.

MANNING, N. (1989) *The Therapeutic Community: Charisma and Routinisation*, London: Routledge.

McMullen, R. (1988) *Living with HIV in Self and Others*, London: Gay Men's Press.

Monette, P. (1988) *Borrowed Time*, London: Collins Harvill.

Money, J. M. (1987) *To All the Girls I've Loved Before*, Boston: Alyson Publications.

Patton, C. (1990) *Inventing AIDS*, London: Routledge.

Small, N. (1993a) *AIDS: the Challenge. Understanding, Education and Care*, Aldershot: Avebury.

Small, N. (1993b) 'HIV/AIDS: Lessons for policy and practice', in D. Clark (Ed.) *The Future of Palliative Care*, Buckingham: Open University Press.

Watney, S. (1994) *Practices of Freedom*, London: Rivers Oram Press.

Chapter 3

Opportunity Lost: HIV/AIDS, Disability and Legislation

Derek Adam-Smith and Fiona Goss

A substantial body of opinion supports the view that the transmission of HIV through everyday work practices is extremely remote. In the limited cases where there is a potential risk, for example in the medical field, this can be controlled by the implementation of specific procedures and hygiene arrangements (Goss and Adam-Smith, 1995). Despite this, evidence suggests that workplace prejudice and discrimination by employers and/or co-workers against people with HIV/AIDS is far from uncommon (Harris and Haigh, 1990; Panos, 1990; Green, 1995; Wilson, 1995). To date, what legal protection exists for employees in the UK against such discrimination has depended on a mishmash of legislation not specifically drawn up with HIV/AIDS in mind. Thus, those with HIV/AIDS in search of protection through current employment law find only limited assistance available. An opportunity to extend protection from employment discrimination to those with HIV was, however, presented by the 1995 Disability Discrimination Act (DDA) whose employment provisions came into force at the end of 1996.[1] Unfortunately this opportunity would seem to have been missed.

We suggest that this failure is associated with the way in which disability has been framed in the Act. It is increasingly recognized that what comes to be seen as 'disability' is partly determined by the many social meanings attached to physical and mental impairments (Oliver, 1990; Shakespeare, 1994). AIDS/HIV in particular raises complex issues involving the interweaving of gender, sexuality, social roles and taboos (Mann, 1995). The implications of these complexities appear largely to have been ignored (intentionally or otherwise) in the drafting of British legislation. Instead of recognizing the existence of a 'social' dimension to discrimination, the government has chosen to use an individualistically based interpretation of disability derived from those adopted by medical practitioners.

This chapter begins by illustrating the types of discrimination to which employees who are HIV-positive have been exposed and for which existing employment law provides limited remedies. Following a brief examination of the ways in which disability may be defined, we consider the aims and provisions of the DDA which we argue is based on an individualistic notion in which disability is seen in terms of a medical phenomenon rather than a social construction. We go on to compare the Act with the approach taken in the 1990 Americans with Disabilities Act (ADA) which, by adopting a more 'social model' of disability, and by presenting discrimination against disabled people as a civil rights issue, offers significantly greater protection for those affected by HIV. We conclude by suggesting that where legal definitions ignore the social dimension of disability, such representation will continue to marginalize the interests of both those employees who are asymptomatic and those who are believed by others to be HIV-positive or have AIDS (but do not).

Discrimination against Employees with HIV/AIDS

While employment is not the only place in which those with HIV/AIDS may be subject to discrimination (Harris and Haigh, 1990) there is a growing body of evidence detailing incidents of workplace discrimination. Wilson (1992) reports that in the experience of HIV-advice agencies, employment problems are the second most common enquiry from their clients. Researchers have also reported a number of cases where employees and potential employees have found their HIV status to be the grounds for discrimination. Green (1995), for example, reports the difficulties that a positive diagnosis presents in gaining and keeping employment and, in particular, the overt discrimination faced as a result of HIV status. These included: (1) a person with haemophilia who went for two job interviews and who noticed a change in the atmosphere immediately he mentioned his HIV status – he was not offered either positions; (2) a teacher who had informed his employer of his HIV status, and who failed to be promoted although he felt he was the most qualified applicant for the post; and (3) a sex worker who was sacked when her colleagues found out that she was HIV-positive and refused to work with her.

Similar evidence emerges from research undertaken by Wilson (1994). She documents a number of cases where the person's seropositivity or the possibility of being HIV-positive lead to loss of employment. These included (1) a building-site labourer whose work colleagues discovered he was a drug user and refused to work with him until he had an HIV test. Before deciding whether or not to take the test he was sacked by the site manager; (2) a person with haemophilia, employed as a wages clerk, whose medical condition was known to his employers. Since his bleeds tended to occur in his knees and ankles he delivered wages to the company's many outlets by car. However, once he was diagnosed as being HIV-positive, this facility was withdrawn and he was required to undertake his deliveries on foot. Severe bleeds followed his first journey and he had some time off work. He was eventually dismissed on grounds of ill-health; and (3) a long-serving supermarket employee who, diagnosed as HIV-positive, agreed with his sympathetic manager to be transferred from work involving cutting machinery. On returning to work after suffering a bout of HIV-related pneumonia he found a new manager in post who made it clear that he wanted the employee to leave. He was transferred to work in the freezer storage room and, after a few months, resigned because of the deterioration of his health caused by his working conditions (Wilson, 1994).

The trigger for discrimination illustrated in these cases is the diagnosis or suspicion of HIV-positive status, irrespective of the possibility that employees may be able to work for many years before their health substantially deteriorates, and that employment can provide a degree of both financial security and self-esteem for those affected. Our own research suggests that such attitudes are formed by a combination of an, often exaggerated, fear of infection and a 'moral distaste' of those who are HIV-positive or who have developed AIDS: the latter is typically accompanied by a level of homophobia (Goss and Adam-Smith, 1995).

Where minority groups are subject to prejudice and unjustifiable discrimination, there are grounds for seeking from the wider society protection in the form of legal redress. In the case of HIV/AIDS, Southam and Howard (1988) argue, for example, that existing sex-discrimination legislation may be applicable in certain circumstances while Harris (1990) identifies situations where such discrimination may fall within the scope of the 1976 Race Relations Act. However, the provisions of these Acts mean that the chances of a successful claim at an industrial tribunal are small and no cases are known to have reached the courts. Equally, the provisions relating to unfair dismissal have been shown, in the small number of cases that have reached the tribunals, to be of limited assistance to those with HIV/AIDS. Indeed, in the majority of these cases the court has supported the employer in finding such dismissals fair. These include a cinema projectionist dismissed when fellow employees feared that toilet facilities might become contaminated with the 'AIDS virus' following the employee's conviction for gross indecency in a public toilet (despite there being no evidence offered that the employee had AIDS or was HIV-positive). Similarly, a ship's cook failed in his claim for unfair redundancy selection after being transferred because co-workers had objected to sailing with him for 'personal hygiene' reasons – the innuendo being that he was gay and thus likely to have HIV (Goss and Adam-Smith, 1995, pp. 132–4).

Thus while existing employment law may provide some assistance for employees discriminated against in circumstances similar to those reported above (Wilson, 1992) the key difficulty often lies in seeking to ensure that the facts of the case fit legal definitions which were not designed specifically to deal with HIV/AIDS. Thus if legislation is to provide adequate protection for those with HIV/AIDS it needs to be drawn in such a way that the forms of discrimination outlined above are made unlawful. Parenthetically, this is not to suggest that simply passing a law will lead to immediate and sustained changes in attitudes. Experience of race and sex discrimination law would caution against such claims (see, for example, Atkins and Hoggert, 1984; O'Donovan, 1985; Fitzpatrick, 1987). There are, however, other compelling grounds in support of a law which provides a positive right of non-discrimination for people with HIV/AIDS. First, and most significantly, such legislation can be seen as a statement by society concerning the kind of behaviour that is un-acceptable and thus enhance the social status of those affected by the disease through a declaration of their civil rights. Second, legal enactment can provide an incentive to employers to develop a constructive approach to people with AIDS, at least as a means of avoiding legal action and, more positively, as an expression of their social responsibility (Belgrave, 1995; Revell, 1995).

In recognition of the limitations of existing law, two attempts were made during the 1980s to introduce specific employment legislation that would give protection to people with HIV/AIDS. The first (drafted by David Alton MP from recommendations made by the Terrence Higgins Trust) sought to make dismissal on the grounds of HIV infection or having AIDS (*or suspicion of this*) an inadmissible reason for dismissal. The second (introduced as an amendment to the 1989 Employment Bill by Gavin Strong MP) attempted to provide a wider scope of protection by making it unlawful to discriminate in the selection of employees, the provision of terms and conditions of employ-ment, and the dismissal of staff on the grounds that the person had con-tracted, *or was believed to be at risk of contracting*, HIV. Although both attempts failed, it was significant that both sought (as the emphasis shows) to introduce the idea that belief of infection was as powerful a source of discrimination as actual seropositivity: a feature that is vital if legislation is to provide pro-tection against HIV-based discrimination. More recently, a further attempt was made to outlaw discrimination against those with HIV/AIDS through the 1994 private member's Civil Rights (Disabled Persons) Bill. Here again, as its title suggests, the Bill recognized a social dimension to the definition of dis-ability which would have provided increased protection to those with HIV/ AIDS. Strongly opposed by the government, the Bill was notoriously 'talked out' in the House of Commons.

Thus with seemingly little likelihood of HIV/AIDS specific employment legislation being enacted, attention has turned to the provisions of the 1995 Disability Discrimination Act. The measure was introduced as the government's response to the adverse publicity attracted by the failure of the Civil Rights Bill to reach the statute book. However, protection for many of those affected by HIV will only be forthcoming if the Act employs a definition that recog-nizes a social construction of disability. The crucial test is, then, the extent to which the definition of disability utilized includes asymptomatic employees, those that might have a 'reputation' of being infected/exposed to HIV as well as those who have developed AIDS. Thus the approach taken by legislators to define disability will be significant in deciding whether or not discrimination on the grounds of HIV/AIDS is covered by the law – and it is to definitional approaches that we now turn.

Definitions of Disability

The way in which people with disabilities have been identified and classified remains a contested area: one that reflects both an historical development and, more significantly, competing ideological perspectives. Definitions of disability are not rationally determined but rather socially constructed: what becomes seen as a disability is determined by the various social meanings attached to certain physical and mental impairments. These may contain the articulated agendas of particular interest groups with potential detrimental effects on people with disabilities as these definitions are used as the basis for the development of social policy. 'The so-called "objective" criteria of disability reflects the biases, self-interests, and moral evaluations of those in a position to influence policy' (Albrecht and Levy, 1981, p. 14). As a result, dominant definitions of 'disability' hold immense power and influence. The crucial determining factor when considering 'disability' as a category is the definitional process: who makes it, why, how and to what intentions is the definition to be put?

In order to illustrate the significance of this process to disability legislation, we consider two broad, but contrasting, approaches: the individualistic and the social. Which approach is adopted reflects in part the objectives of, and balance of power between, competing interest groups.

Individualistic definitions locate the problems of disability with the person: the difficulties disabled people face are a direct result of their 'individual physical, sensory or intellectual impairments' (French, 1994, p. 3). These individualistic definitions depend on a distinction between an impairment (an organically based disturbance in bodily structure) and disability, referring to the individual's inability to perform the major functions of 'normal' daily living as a result of their 'individual impairment'. Disability is thus most usually viewed 'in terms of disease process, abnormality and personal tragedy' (French, 1994, p. 3). This approach is most explicitly demonstrated by medical definitions of disability and has dominated clinical practice and policy.[2] Such an approach tends to support the *status quo* since: 'the sub-normality of the individual rather than the sub-normality of the environment, tends to be blamed for any inadequacies' (Ryan and Thomas, 1987, p. 27).

With respect to HIV/AIDS medical professionals have:

> remained essentially focused on the physical dimensions of health. In the biomedical mode of thinking we have thought more about disease, disability and death than well being. (Mann, 1995, p. 44)

The adoption of individualistically based frameworks has placed the response to, and treatment of, HIV/AIDS in a situation where narrow medical perspectives fail to confront social inequalities associated with the disease. For example, in terms of vulnerability to acquiring HIV infection, those who are currently marginalized, stigmatized and discriminated against will be the ones most likely to be affected by the pandemic in the future. Thus a failure to take account of the wider social and economic disadvantages surrounding potential HIV infection places a substantial limitation on the possible action available to overcome discrimination. Further, by seeking to contain the definition (and by implication the solution) within a narrow medical term, such an approach suggests that 'normal' is an absolute category. 'Normality' becomes the yardstick against which (dis)ability is judged and consequently this approach 'imposes an assumption of biological inferiority upon disabled individuals' (Hahn, 1986, p. 131). People with disabilities, people with HIV/AIDS, will be required to conform to society's norms, a process which fails to take account of differing social and cultural contexts.[3]

In contrast to the individualistic, the 'social' approach to disability uses a definition deriving from the belief that the problems disabled people face come not from their physical or mental limitations but from an 'inappropriate social response to them' (Hasler, 1993, p. 280). Problems of disability are seen here not within the individual but within society. Such a belief has developed from within the ideas of people with disabilities themselves and stem from their unhappiness with professional practice and the wider discrimination faced from society. This approach suggests that the problems of disability are thus largely located in society's response to impairment.[4] The view that society disables challenges the 'very assumption of normality', where disabled people are excluded from everyday life by not being able to read the gas bill, by lack of access to public buildings, by being denied a means of making a living:

> Being disabled is a reflection of the power relationship that segregates some members of society by organizing the environment only around the needs of able-bodied members. (Appleby, 1994, p. 19)

As a result, people with disabilities experience specific oppression. Seen from this perspective, disability becomes an issue of civil rights, not a problem located within the individual.

The issue of civil rights has significant resonance for those with HIV/ AIDS where perceptions of 'normality' are merged with the (perhaps hidden) agenda underlying the definitional process. Where a traditional sense of social identity sees abnormal as 'not like us' and unashamed social 'deviants' such as gay men and injecting drug users as objects of threat and repulsion, ostracism and discrimination can be justified by those who are 'normal' (Goss and Adam-Smith, 1995; Marquet, Hubert and Campenhoudt, 1995). The early characterization of HIV/AIDS as the 'gay plague' has meant that it carries with it a constant reference to homosexuality (Watney, 1989; Weeks, 1991) and the conflation of AIDS and homosexuality may lead to a strong moral outrage at suggestions of offering protection from discrimination for those with AIDS. Such views can be illustrated by the reaction of sections of the media and pressure groups representing 'normal social values' to the successful amendment to the then Disability Discrimination Bill which included symptomatic HIV within the meaning of disability. Carrying the story under a front-page banner headline, 'Storm over AIDS victims', the *Daily Mail* reported that the government had accepted the amendment rather than retain their original intention of 'confining any reference to AIDS or its symptoms to regulations associated with the Bill' (Eastham, 1995, p. 2). Commenting on the 'uproar' caused by the move, the newspaper summarized objections by Tory MPs and family campaigners who:

> strenuously oppose putting AIDS suffers [sic], who in this country mainly contract the illness from homosexual relations or sharing contaminated drug needles, on a par with the disabled who did nothing to contract their affliction.

The report (Eastham, 1995, p. 2) goes on to quote Dr Adrian Rogers, director of the Conservative Family Institute, as saying: 'It's crazy. People who behave morally do not get AIDS, full stop.' Attempts to restrict or widen the definition of disability and thus the extent to which it will encompass HIV status will not, as the above discussion illustrates, be a matter of rational logic but the result of a political process not divorced from moral judgments.

Approaching Disability: the UK and USA Compared

The legal definition of disability is important since it will determine who is protected by legislation. In doing so definitions can maintain the view that disability is a problem for the individual (and, by definition, so is the solution) or approach disability as a social construct resulting from the person's location in a wider social and physical environment. From the latter perspective, people have impairments but society disables.

The manner in which these two approaches underpin legal provisions can be seen through a comparison of the 1995 United Kingdom's Disability Discrimination Act (DDA) and the 1990 Americans with Disabilities Act (ADA). The choice of comparators is particularly apposite since the Civil Rights (Disabled Persons) Bill, the failed Private Member's Bill, was heavily modelled on the American Act and might therefore have been expected to achieve the same objectives.

At first sight both the DDA and the ADA contain a number of similarities. Both extend legal redress to people with disabilities who suffer discrimination in employment (and other aspects of social life including discrimination in the provision of goods and services). Both contain provisions making discrimination unlawful in matters such as recruitment, pay and other terms of employment, promotion and dismissal if these are shown to be on the basis of disability. Both require employers to take action to facilitate the employment or continued employment of disabled people, termed 'reasonable accommodation' in the ADA and 'reasonable adjustment' in the DDA. Both concede that in determining what is 'reasonable' action, its cost in relation to the financial resources of the employer is to be taken into consideration. Both, in what may be seen as a reinforcement of the last point, provide an exemption for small firms: employers with less than fifteen employees in the case of the ADA and those with fewer than twenty in the UK are exempt from the law's requirements. However, beneath the superficial similarity there are fundamental differences in the aims of the two pieces of legislation and this can be seen in the origins of their respective definitions of disability. We consider the aims and purposes of the two pieces of legislation since these will indicate the scope intended by the measures and the governments' commitment to the removal of discrimination against disabled people, and, in relation to this, the definitions of disability used. In doing so, we suggest that while the UK Act draws its definitions from individualized models of disability, the American approach recognizes the role of the wider society in '(dis)abling' those with physical or mental impairments. We argue therefore that while there is limited room for some optimism, as currently constructed the UK Act holds little by way of protection for those with HIV.

In its preamble to the Act the ADA notes that:

> individuals with disabilities are a discrete and insular minority who have been faced with restrictions and limitations, subject to a history of purposeful unequal treatment, and relegated to a position of political powerlessness in our society, based on characteristics that are beyond the control of such individuals and resulting from stereotypic assumptions not truly indicative of the individual ability of such individuals to participate in, and contribute to, society. (ADA 2(a)(7))

The purposes of the Act are then set out, which are designed to outlaw such discriminatory treatment against people with disabilities. These include providing a clear and comprehensive national mandate for the elimination of discrimination against individuals with disabilities; providing clear, strong, consistent, enforceable standards addressing discrimination against individuals with disabilities; ensuring that the Federal government plays a central role in enforcing the standards established in this Act on behalf of individuals with disabilities; and invoking the sweep of congressional authority in order to address the major areas of discrimination faced day-to-day by people with disabilities (ADA, 1990, 2(b)).

The Act thus provides a clear signal of the US government's intentions. It recognizes that people with disabilities are a minority group whose relative lack of power has not allowed them to achieve fair and equal treatment in the face of prejudice from society, and that this can only be achieved if there is a commitment by the government to use its legal powers in support of the elimination of discrimination. While accepting that their achievement requires more than the passing of a piece of legislation, the Act offers a clear declaration of the civil rights of people with disabilities (Pfeiffer, 1994).

The apparent rationale for the DDA can be discerned in the negative stance taken by the UK government to the Civil Rights (Disabled Persons) Bill. In opposing this Bill it clearly indicated that, unlike its American counterpart, the foundation of civil rights for disabled people through the establishment of legislation was not part of the government's agenda. During the House of Commons debate on the Bill, the then government minister with responsibility for disabled people: 'reiterated the government view that it failed to take account of the interests of the business fraternity, and that the cost of implementation would prove far too expensive' (Barnes and Oliver, 1995, p. 112). The implication here is that in addition to the (disputed) high cost of implementing its provisions, the needs of business should take priority over the needs of people with disabilities: a view reinforced in the preface to the government's paper on discrimination against disabled people: 'We must move forward, within a realistic timetable, with practical measures to tackle discrimination *which also take account of the potential impact on employers*' (EDDP, 1995, p. 3, with emphasis added).

On the specific matter of costs, however, Pfeiffer (1994) argues that the ADA embodies a series of cost-containment measures that tend to limit the expenditure necessary to conform to the requirements of the Act, questioning the government's objection to the Civil Rights Bill in terms of the financial burden it would place on business. It is interesting to note that in his first speech as a Labour MP, Alan Howarth, who 'crossed the floor', chose to take issue with the government's objections to the Bill. He argued that when the benefits that flowed from the Bill were taken into account, the net cost would have been nil (Howarth, 1995).

Defining Disability: the UK Approach

Both the ADA and the DDA refer to the protection of people with disabilities and thus the crucial issue is the protected class of people – what is meant by 'disability' and who is covered as far as the two measures are concerned? In the UK, the DDA states that:

> a person has a disability for the purposes of this Act if he has a physical or mental impairment which has a substantial and long-term adverse effect on his ability to carry out normal day-to-day activities. (DDA, 1995, Section 2)

Physical impairments are not elaborated on in the Act except that they must affect normal day-to-day activities defined as mobility; manual dexterity; physical coordination; continence; ability to lift, carry or otherwise move everyday objects; speech, hearing or eyesight; memory, or ability to learn, understand or concentrate; or perception of the risk of danger. The Minister for Social Security and Disabled People has stated that:

> *The list is intended to be exhaustive* in the sense that, taken together, the capabilities listed provide sufficient indication for users of the legislation and the courts of what impairments the Bill is designed to cover. (Quoted in IRS, 1995, p. 27, with emphasis added)

Mental impairments are included '*only if the illness is a clinically well-recognized illness*' (DDA, Sch 1(1)) which according to the minister refers to a 'reasonably substantial *body of practitioners* who accept that the condition exists' (IRS, 1995, p. 16, with emphasis added in both citations).

Through a prescribed list of impairments, the DDA definition locates disability as a problem for the individual and thus draws heavily on non-social models of disability. This approach is reinforced in the medicalization of mental impairments which will only satisfy the legal definition if medical practitioners are able to confirm the existence of the illness or condition. This formulation of the definition of disability echoes those based on a model of disability which sees it as an individual issue (French, 1994). In reviewing the problems associated with the Act, Barnes and Oliver (1995, p. 113) argue that it: 'is firmly rooted in the medical rather than the social model of disability. It sets out to prohibit discrimination against disabled people on the grounds of their (not society's) disability.' Thus employers may be tempted not to recruit or dismiss people they believe might acquire legal protection at some stage in the future.

We suggest that there are likely to be practical difficulties in establishing who does and who does not come within the protection of the Act. Under Schedule 1 (8), those who have developed AIDS will apparently be protected by the Act's provisions once the onset of the progressive condition has an effect on their day-to-day activities, even if the effect is not 'substantial'. However, the position of those with asymptomatic HIV, or those believed to be so by others, is very different: their condition would not meet the (medical) definition of an impairment, thus allowing employers to dismiss or not recruit people they believe might acquire legal protection at some stage in the future. As we show below, the definition used by the ADA, being much more widely drawn, will more readily encompass those who have not developed AIDS-related illnesses.

In contrast to the DDA, the ADA provides a broad three-pronged definition of disability. With respect to an individual, this means a physical or mental impairment that substantially limits one or more of the major life activities of such individual; a record of such impairments; and being regarded as having such an impairment (ADA, 1990, 3(2)). Unlike the DDA, there is no attempt within the Act to list possible disabilities. Similarly, while regulations produced under the ADA define physical and mental impairments, 'the temptation to list exhaustively the kinds of conditions which will be counted as impairments is . . . resisted in the regulations' (Doyle, 1995, p. 94).

In relation to HIV, particular significance can be attached to the wording used to define the impact of an impairment. While the DDA refers to *normal day-to-day activities*, the latter takes a wider, more open approach. While offering *examples* of what may be considered to be a major life activity (which are not too dissimilar to those of the UK Act) the more generalized approach of the ADA allows for other activities to be included. Indeed, the ADA specifically notes that:

> a person infected with the Human Immunodeficiency Virus is covered under the first prong of the definition of the term 'disability' because of a substantial limitation to procreation and intimate sexual relationships. (ADA, 1990, p. 52)

For those with HIV/AIDS there are, then, significant differences in the result of the definitions used by the two pieces of legislation. Under the ADA, those with both symptomatic and asymptomatic HIV are covered. In the UK, those who have developed AIDS would appeared to be covered (although there is some indication that the government would have preferred as little publicity as possible of this fact) but those who have not developed illnesses which have an effect on their day-to-day activities (as defined) will enjoy no protection from employment discrimination.

Although the ADA's provisions encompass HIV-positive people, it is important to note that concern over HIV status has lead to an apparent anomaly in the Act. An amendment introduced during its passage allows employers to discriminate against disabled people who have a (listed) infectious disease which is transmittable through food-handling. The amendment was promoted because of concern in the catering industry that employing known or 'suspected' HIV-positive people might lead to loss of business through customer boycott (despite there being no evidence that the virus is transmissible through food-handling). As Doyle (1995, p. 102) notes:

> This is a curious example of a particular provision in a statute, generally designed to eliminate discrimination based upon ignorance, being shaped by a desire to accommodate misunderstanding.

Despite this particular provision, the ADA provides much stronger protection for those with AIDS than the UK Bill. This can be illustrated by examining other differences in the approach taken towards disability by the two governments – a difference which Doyle (1995) points out is shown in the ADA's admission of a social construction of disability. This is most obvious, and of specific relevance to the issue of HIV/AIDS, in the third definition of disability under the Act: 'being regarded as having such an impairment'. A person regarded as having an impairment is one who (1) has a physical or mental impairment that does not substantially limit major life activities but that is treated . . . as constituting such a limitation; (2) has a physical or mental impairment that substantially limits major life activities only as a result of the attitudes of others towards such impairment; or (3) has none of the impairments defined (. . . .) but is treated (. . . .) as having such an impairment (cited in Doyle, 1995, p. 175).

The justification for such a definition is contained in the recital of Congressional hearings contained within the Act which drew attention to the impact of society's myths and fears about disease and disability:

> A person who is excluded from any basic life activity, or is otherwise discriminated against, because of [an employer's] negative attitudes towards that impairment is treated as having a disability. Thus, for example, if an employer refuses to hire someone because of a fear of the 'negative reactions' of others to the individual or because of the employer's perception that the applicant has an impairment which prevents that person from working, that person is covered under the third prong of the definition of disability. (ADA, 1990, p. 53)

Thus discrimination based on stereotypes and prejudice, both of which are characteristic of society's attitudes to HIV/AIDS, are caught under the Act. Indeed, as we noted above, although eschewing a list of conditions that will be considered as impairments, the legislators specifically included infection with HIV as an illustration of what might be included. Thus under the ADA, discrimination by an employer against an employee or applicant which is based on the *belief* that the person might be HIV-positive would also be unlawful. In the UK, by contrast, those who may be *perceived* as being HIV-positive are not covered by any of the Act's provisions. In specifically rejecting inclusion of belief of HIV-positive status, the Minister for Social Security and Disabled People indicated that the government had no intention of broadening the definitions of disability:

> I do not think that we could justify to the country including in the [Act] *people who were thought to have HIV* (. . . .) Including people who were thought to be HIV would make the terms of the [Act] much broader because it would apply to people other than those who have disabilities or who are *understood to be disabled* in any generally accepted sense of the term. (Quoted in IRS, 1995, p. 28, with emphasis added)

This view confirms the intention to maintain a narrow definition of disability and to provide protection only to those who are seen to be 'genuinely' disabled and thus 'deserving of society's compassion'.

There is one further aspect of the ADA which marks out the difference between it and the DDA, and which has potential implications for AIDS-related discrimination. The ADA acknowledges the possibility of 'discrimination by association' in Section 2 (b)(4) which prohibits discrimination by an employer (by excluding or otherwise denying access to equal jobs or benefits) against an individual who has a relationship or association with a person who has a known disability. Since this protection is not limited to those who have a familial relationship with the disabled individual, it would seem that in the context of HIV/AIDS this would prohibit employment discrimination against a person caring for, or living with, someone with AIDS. This possibility was made known to the Congressional Committee in testimony concerning a long-serving female employee who was dismissed when her employer discovered that her son, who had become ill with an AIDS-related condition, had moved into her home so that she could care for him (ADA, 1990, p. 30). The ADA thus provides a high level of protection for those who are asymptomatic, have developed AIDS or who have a relationship with someone who is HIV-positive or developed AIDS, or where there is a perception that the person may be HIV-positive.

Conclusions

AIDS is a relatively new phenomenon, but those infected with HIV are already hallmarked with high levels of intolerance underpinned by 'moral' judgements and particular attitudes towards sexuality. The workplace is one such arena in which discrimination can occur, be it from employers or work colleagues. The cases reported at the beginning of this chapter illustrate the consequences for the individual of prejudicial behaviour. However, as we have explored, the passing of the DDA in the UK will do nothing to help the majority of employees who find themselves in similar positions, whereas if these incidents had occurred in the USA disability legislation would have provided protection.

Definitions of disability which draw on models which locate disability as an individual problem will only provide marginal help to people with disabilities, including those with HIV/AIDS. As Oliver (1990) argues, people will behave in response to the meanings given to objects in the social world. Thus:

As far as disability is concerned, if it is seen as a tragedy, then disabled people will be treated as if they are the victims of some tragic happening or circumstance. This treatment (will be) . . . translated into social policies which will attempt to compensate these victims for the tragedies that have befallen them. Alternatively . . . if disability is defined as social oppression, then disabled people will be seen as the collective victims of an uncaring or unknowing society

> rather than as individual victims of circumstance. Such a view will be
> translated into social policies geared towards alleviating oppression
> rather than compensating individuals. (Oliver, 1990, p. 2)

However, those with HIV/AIDS are not seen by many in society as being affected by a tragic, undeserved event but rather infection with the virus is perceived to be the consequence of a self-induced affliction resulting from immoral and repugnant behaviour associated with a perverted lifestyle. This view thus questions whether such people are even deserving of sympathy let alone compensation (see, for example, Goss and Adam-Smith, 1995). Discrimination against those with AIDS can be seen as a form of social oppression requiring the formal establishment of their civil rights.

This cannot be done by legislation alone: the law is more effective when seeking to deal with problems that arise as a result of discrimination than it is in trying to deal with its causes. However, as the Americans with Disabilities Act shows, treating disability as socially constructed, combined with a clear commitment to address the discrimination that flows from this, can provide a foundation on which civil rights can develop. We contend that in the absence of a similar commitment among law-makers in the UK, those with HIV (and those with many other disabilities) will remain marginalized and be denied even this building block of social justice and self-esteem.

Notes

1   Part III of the Act aims to make unlawful discrimination against people with disabilities in the provision of goods, facilities and services. These provisions are expected to be phased in over a number of years.

2   Many definitions of disability in use are based around a medical model of disability. These definitions are often unchallenged by 'professionals' dealing with disabled people. The World Health Organization's (WHO) is one such definition. Here, impairment is defined as any loss or abnormality of psychological, physiological or anatomical structure or function; disability is seen as any restriction or lack of ability (resulting from an impairment) to perform an activity in the manner or within the range considered normal for a human being; and handicap is viewed as disadvantage for a given individual, resulting from an impairment or disability, that limits or prevents the fulfilment of a role (depending on age, sex and social and cultural factors) for that individual (Massie, 1994, p. 5).

3   Approaching disability from an individualistic perspective has produced an interesting development that may encourage self-identification among people with disabilities as a distinct social group or groups. The sharing of a common identity can stimulate debate among those with disabilities over the discrimination to which they are exposed (Finklestein, 1993). Such alliances can be seen in the emergence

of pressure groups working for improved social and welfare provisions for those with HIV/AIDS (Harris and Haigh, 1990; Cowan, 1995; Nicholson, 1995).

4   Impairment is the lack of part or all of a limb, or having a defective limb, organ or mechanism of the body. Disability is the loss or limitation of opportunities that prevents people who have impairments from taking part in the normal life of the community on an equal level with others because of physical and social barriers (Finkelstein and French, 1993).

References

ALBRECHT, G. and LEVY, J. (1981) 'Constructing disabilities as social problems', in G. ALBRECHT (Ed.) *Cross National Rehabilitation Policies: A Sociological Perspective*, London: Sage.

APPLEBY, Y. (1994) 'Out in the margins', *Disability and Society*, **9**, 1, pp. 19–32.

ATKINS, S. and HOGGERT, B. (1984) *Women and the Law*, Oxford: Blackwell.

BARNES, C. and OLIVER, M. (1995) 'Disability rights: rhetoric and reality in the UK', *Disability and Society*, **10**, 1, pp. 111–16.

BELGRAVE, S. (1995) 'One employer's approach to employee education', in D. FITZSIMMONS, V. HARDY and K. TOLLEY (Eds) *Socio-Economic Impact of AIDS in Europe*, London: Cassell.

COWAN, D. (1995) 'HIV and homelessness: intervention and backlash in local authority policy', in D. FITZSIMMONS, V. HARDY and K. TOLLEY (Eds) *Socio-Economic Impact of AIDS in Europe*, London: Cassell.

DOYLE, B. (1995) *Disability, Discrimination and Equal Opportunities: A Comparative Study of the Employment Rights of Disabled Persons*, London: Mansell.

EASTHAM, P. (1995) 'Storm over AIDS victims', *Daily Mail*, 28 August.

EDDP (1995) *Ending Discrimination Against Disabled People*, London: HMSO.

FINKLESTEIN, V. (1993) 'The commonality of disability', in J. SWAIN, V. FINKLESTEIN, S. FRENCH and M. OLIVER (Eds) *Disabling Barriers – Enabling Environments*, London: Sage.

FINKLESTEIN, V. and FRENCH, S. (1993) 'Towards a psychology of disability', in J. SWAIN, V. FINKLESTEIN, S. FRENCH and M. OLIVER (Eds) *Disabling Barriers – Enabling Environments*, London: Sage.

FITZPATRICK, P. (1987) 'Racism and the innocence of law', *Journal of Legal Studies*, **14**, 1, pp. 119–32.

FRENCH, S. (1994) *On Equal Terms – Working with Disabled People*, Oxford: Butterworth-Heinemann.

GOSS, D. and ADAM-SMITH, D. (1995) *Organizing AIDS: Workplace and Organizational Responses to the HIV/AIDS Epidemic.* London: Taylor & Francis.

GREEN, G. (1995) 'Processes of stigmatization and impact on employment of people with HIV', in D. FITZSIMMONS, V. HARDY and K. TOLLEY (Eds) *Socio-Economic Impact of AIDS in Europe*, London: Cassell.

HAHN, H. (1986) 'Public support for rehabilitation programs: the analysis of US disability policy, disability', *Handicap and Society*, **1**, 2, pp. 121–37.

HARRIS, D. (1990) 'AIDS and employment', in D. HARRIS and R. HAIGH (Eds) *AIDS: A Guide to the Law*, London: Routledge.

HARRIS, D. and HAIGH, R. (1990) (Eds) *AIDS: A Guide to the Law*, London: Routledge.

HASLER, F. (1993) 'Developments in the disabled people's movement', in J. SWAIN, V. FINKLESTEIN, S. FRENCH and M. OLIVER (Eds) *Disabling Barriers – Enabling Environments*, London: Sage.

HOWARTH, A. (1995) 'Disabled and denied', *Guardian*, 23 October.

IRS (1995) 'The Disability Discrimination Bill', *Equal Opportunities Review*, March/April.

MANN, J. (1995) 'AIDS, health and human rights: the future of the pandemic', *RSA Journal*, August/September, pp. 40–8.

MARQUET, J., HUBERT, M. and CAMPENHOUDT, L. (1995) 'Public awareness of AIDS: discrimination and the effects of mistrust', in D. FITZSIMMONS, V. HARDY and K. TOLLEY (Eds) *Socio-Economic Impact of AIDS in Europe*, London: Cassell.

MASSIE, B. (1994) *Disabled People and Social Justice*, London: IPPR.

NICHOLSON, J. (1995) 'Back to basics: securing funding for voluntary HIV services', in D. FITZSIMMONS, V. HARDY and K. TOLLEY (Eds) *Socio-Economic Impact of AIDS in Europe*, London: Cassell.

O'DONOVAN, K. (1985) *Sexual Divisions in the Law*, London: Weidenfeld & Nicholson.

OLIVER, M. (1990) *The Politics of Disablement*, Basingstoke: Macmillan.

PANOS (1990) *The Third Epidemic: Repercussions of the Fear of AIDS*, London: Panos.

PFEIFFER, D. (1994) 'The Americans with Disabilities Act: costly mandate or civil rights?', *Disability and Society*, **9**, 4, pp. 533–42.

REVELL, A. (1995) 'Wellcome's positive action in response to HIV and AIDS', in D. FITZSIMMONS, V. HARDY and K. TOLLEY (Eds) *Socio-Economic Impact of AIDS in Europe*, London: Cassell.

RYAN, J. and THOMAS, F. (1987) *The Politics of Mental Handicap*, London: Free Association Books.

SHAKESPEARE, T. (1994) 'Cultural representations of disabled people: dustbins for disavowal?', *Disability and Society*, **9**, 3. pp. 283–99.

SOUTHAM, C. and HOWARD, G. (1988) *AIDS and Employment Law*, London: Financial Training Publications.

WATNEY, S. (1989) 'The subject of AIDS', in P. AGGLETON, G. HART and P. DAVIES (Eds) *AIDS: Social Representations, Social Practices*, Lewes: Falmer Press.

WEEKS, J. (1991) *Against Nature*, London: Rivers Oram Press.

WILSON, P. (1992) *HIV and AIDS in the Workplace*, London: National AIDS Trust.

WILSON, P. (1994) 'Colleague or viral vector? The legal construction of the HIV-positive worker', *Law and Policy*, Fall issue, **16**, 3, pp. 299–321.

WILSON, P. (1995) 'Discrimination in the workplace: protection and the law in the UK', in D. FITZSIMMONS, V. HARDY and K. TOLLEY (Eds) *Socio-Economic Impact of AIDS*, London: Cassell.

Chapter 4

AIDS Policy Communities in Australia

Mark Edwards

HIV/AIDS impacts on groups that have traditionally been viewed as marginal and diffuse, including gay men, injecting drug users (IDUs), sex workers and people with haemophilia. According to the traditional medical-based approach to health policy, such marginalized groups would have had minimal success in gaining access to adequate care and humane treatment. Yet in Australia the groups in society most affected by the disease have achieved considerable success in obtaining health care and access to education and prevention, as well as social support in the form of positive government-funded publicity and legal sanctions outlawing discrimination on the grounds of actual or assumed HIV infection. That this has occurred in a climate of fiscal constraint makes the success of HIV/AIDS communities even more striking.

HIV/AIDS is the first infectious disease to enter consciousness through the media, initially through the gay media and later through the mainstream press. The way the media has reported HIV/AIDS clearly illustrates the reasons for the development of a community-based response to the disease; it also indicates the hostile political and social environment which existed during the early 1980s.

With the emergence of AIDS during 1983, the gay male community in Australia mobilized itself very quickly, effectively engaging the skills and contacts developed during the previous decade of gay political activism. The gay press and the infant AIDS action committees (often one and the same) shared information on AIDS and acted as the only conduit of information and advice to the gay community more generally.

Australia's experience of HIV differs from that of other industrialized nations. The groups most affected by the virus in Australia are gay men, IDUs, sex workers and those infected through medical procedures. Yet in the US, for instance, affected groups also include Haitians (prominent only in the early years of the epidemic) and urban heterosexuals, predominantly African–Americans. AIDS is now the number one cause of death for all Americans in the mid-20 to mid-30 age group. Scotland has yet another experience, as HIV infection there is largely confined to IDUs. The important point is that, despite differing experiences at the international level, HIV/AIDS remains an issue for those groups and individuals already marginalized in the industrialized nations.

More than One Epidemic?

There is acceptance of the notion of not one, but many, AIDS epidemics in Australia. The *Report of the Evaluation of the National HIV/AIDS Strategy* (1992, p. 15) stated that 'the spread of HIV in Australia must be considered as a number of separate, though interrelated epidemics'. Watson (1993, p. 5) concurs with this approach, noting that the full extent of the disease 'can only be appreciated if each of these separate epidemics is examined on its own'. The largest group which has been infected with the virus are 'men who have sex with men' which includes men who identify as homosexual, gay, bisexual and those who may not identify with any of these categories but who still have sex with men. In December 1994 this category accounted for some 85 per cent of all known HIV infections in Australia – and of these 3 per cent were also IDUs.

Before 1985 (when the routine testing of all blood donations commenced), people with medically acquired HIV/AIDS were the second largest group of HIV infected people in Australia. It is estimated that some 430 people have become infected through exposure to infected blood or infected blood products. The issue of medically acquired AIDS continues to be a controversial social and legal one, particularly as it relates to the questions of medical negligence and financial compensation. The principal social impact of medical transmission of the virus is the perpetuation of the notions of 'innocent' and 'guilty' victims.

Australian experience with IDUs differs greatly from overseas experience because Australian data shows much lower rates of infection among this population. Infection rates have been comparatively low (about 5 per cent of the total infected population). The early introduction of needle-exchange programmes in Australia may have slowed the rate of new infections in this group. Watson (1993) notes that ignorance of HIV risk among young occasional injecting amphetamine users may result in a 'future explosion' of HIV in IDUs.

Transmission via heterosexual sex follows a similar pattern to that of IDUs. Infection rates in this group have been low (national surveillance figures in December 1994 indicate that 7 per cent of all HIV infections in Australia were attributed to heterosexual sex). However, the evidence suggests there is a gradual increase in the annual rate of infection in the heterosexual population. In the industrialized nations, several studies have shown that sex work is not a major risk factor in HIV transmission, except where the sex worker also injects drugs. 'It is not clear in all cases whether this is due to safer behaviour on the part of sex workers or to low prevalence of HIV among their clients' (Crofts, 1992, p. 45). Low rates among heterosexual adults, together with equally low rates among IDUs, mean there are very few cases of maternal–infant transmission of HIV in Australia.

Communities: Policy Communities/AIDS Communities

AIDS community-based organizations (CBOs) claim to represent those communities infected with and affected by HIV. Yet the question remains in many people's minds: exactly whom do they represent? As Altman (1990, p. 16) observes:

> We might note at the outset that 'community based organisation' is itself a problematic term, which in practice has caused considerable political problems. Some of the AIDS Councils were founded quite explicitly by public meetings called by already existing gay organisations; all of them have had to grapple with the question as to how far they have a particular relationship to the gay/lesbian community (itself a term of some consternation). The development of specific organisations for sex workers, IV drug users and People (Living) with AIDS suggests that even those Councils which claim to be all inclusive are not perceived as able to fully represent all these groups.

So what is a community? More importantly, what is an HIV/AIDS community? The late Robert Ariss, a former convenor of People Living with AIDS (PLWAs, now known as PLWHAs) raised the notion of 'community' in a paper given to the 4th Australian National AIDS Conference in 1990. He stated that in relation to HIV/AIDS, the term 'community' most obviously refers to 'people with HIV and AIDS'. He went on to note that 'community' can also refer to:

> our friends, lovers and carers, our families; it can also refer to those involved in AIDS professionally, including health care and service workers, educators and AIDS bureaucrats. It refers to those who choose to remain outside formal structures – the activists; and it includes a professional class we rely on in a very immediate, literally life and death way – physicians and researchers who develop and provide treatment for HIV infection. (Cited in van Reyk, 1990, p. 15)

From a public policy perspective, such a grouping of individuals and organizations could be classified as a policy community, a segment of the political system which:

> acquires a dominant voice in determining government decisions in a specific field of public policy, and is generally permitted by society at large and the public authorities in particular to determine public policy in that field. It is populated by government agencies, pressure groups, media people, and individuals, including academics, who have interest in a particular policy field and attempt to influence it. (Pross, 1986, p. 98)

The operation of policy communities has been observed in Britain (Jordan, 1981) and in Canada (Pross, 1986); the concept appears to be equally applicable to policy-making in Australia in the 1980s and the early 1990s. Davis, Wanna and Warhurst *et al.* (1988) identify policy communities operating in Australia in the fields of industrial relations, agriculture, education and ex-service issues. According to Davis, Wanna and Warhurst *et al.* (1988, p. 95), a policy community 'shares a commitment to policies, programs and ways of doing things'. Further, it is argued that members of a policy community agree on the 'survival of the existing arrangements' (Davis, Wanna and Warhurst, 1988, p. 96). To what extent does this analysis hold true in relation to HIV/AIDS policy in Australia? While a degree of cohesion can be identified in the AIDS field, there are a substantial number of variations in the approach taken by groups operating in the field in Australia. Different and sometimes competing groups often promulgate differing, and often conflicting, objectives and policy directions. Therefore, in the Australian context it is more correct to talk of several AIDS policy communities, rather than just one.

The Australian Response: The Emergence of a Community Response

Australia's first community-based AIDS organization, the AIDS Action Committee in NSW, was established in mid-1983 in response to the first reported cases of AIDS in Australia. In August 1984, members of the gay community attending the 9th National Conference of Lesbians and Homosexual Men formed the Australian AIDS Action Committee – the first national community-based organization, which later developed into the Australian Federation of AIDS Organizations (AFAO). Following that conference, members of this new committee met with Neal Blewett, the Federal Minister for Health. 'The national response to HIV/AIDS had begun' (Keenan and van Reyk, 1993, p. 2).

In November 1984 it was announced that four babies had died in Queensland after being infected with contaminated blood donated by a gay man. The Queensland National Party attempted to link the Australian Labor Party (ALP) with the promotion of homosexuality. The federal health minister quickly responded by establishing two national advisory bodies – one medical, the other community-based. A National Health and Medical Research Council (NH&MRC) working party became the AIDS Task Force with the mission to provide scientific advice to all health ministers. The National Advisory Committee on AIDS (NACAIDS) was established to provide a dialogue between the Commonwealth and the communities affected (Gray, 1987, p. 234). The death of what came to be known as the Queensland babies could have had devastating effects on the gay community through a public backlash blaming the death of the children directly on gay men in general. Yet this incident worked to the advantage of the gay community by galvanizing the gay community 'and everybody else for the next phase of the epidemic' (Carr, 1992, p. 17).

In May 1987 the government launched its first national education strategy, the now infamous 'Grim Reaper' campaign. It soon became obvious that it was doomed to failure as its target audience, the general community, was not really a community at risk. The following year both NACAIDS and the Task Force were abolished and replaced by the National Council on AIDS (ANCA), composed of seven medical and eight non-medical members. This move focused attention on contemporary conflict about health care models – the medico-scientific and a more community-oriented one. It is commonly thought that the community-based approach has triumphed in the Australian response to HIV/AIDS. The government believed that involving community groups 'recognises the value of peer education, and the public health benefit of encouraging the people most affected by AIDS to co-operate with the Government in dealing with the problem – rather than alienating or punishing them' (Howe, 1992, p. 2).

In August 1989 the Commonwealth launched a national response to HIV/AIDS in the form of the National HIV/AIDS Strategy. This approach favoured the implementation of a partnership which emphasized community participation and consultation. The Australian response to HIV/AIDS has therefore emphasized the role of community-based organizations. The National Strategy, as devised by the Commonwealth and endorsed by all state and territory governments, provided mechanisms for community involvement; and continued Commonwealth funding has given the policy real meaning. As a result of the Strategy, community-based organizations have 'come to argue for a right to representation in all arenas where policies are established, setting precedents for community representation in a number of institutions which go beyond normal Australian practice' (Altman, 1993, p. 7).

In October 1993 the Commonwealth, in association with all state and territory governments, announced that the National Strategy would be continued for the period 1993–94 to 1995–96. While continuing the general thrust of the first strategy period, the Commonwealth signalled consideration of mainstreaming of HIV/AIDS programmes and activities, as well as the possibility of variations in programme emphasis between the various states and territories.

Explaining Community Involvement

The gay male community accounts for approximately 85 per cent of those infected with HIV, and the same group remains the one that is most at risk of new infections. Thus, gay men form the largest single identifiable group in the community affected by HIV/AIDS. During the course of the epidemic, it has been observed that 'gay leaders have moved from an anarchistic revolutionary politics in the 1970s to a professional, bureaucratised politics in the 1980s' (Plummer, 1988, p. 42). This may in part explain the success of gay community representatives in the HIV/AIDS policy process. The skills acquired by members of the gay community have certainly placed them in a relatively advantageous position to deal with a crisis such as AIDS. 'Building upon human rights movements of the 1960s and 1970s, gay men were able to organise politically and financially in such a way that less cohesive groups at risk, such as intravenous drug users (IVDUs) were not' (Aron, 1991, p. 489).

Another possible explanation for the incorporation of community groups into HIV/AIDS policy-making in Australia was the consensus-generating policy processes adopted by the federal Australian Labor Party government elected in 1983, together with the existence of several 'friendly' ALP governments at the state level. Blewett commented on the style of decision-making under Prime Minister Hawke, stating:

> Given the exceptional willingness of the states to surrender to the Commonwealth a role in health delivery in exchange for resources and access to US expertise, HIV presented a rare opportunity for the exercise of political will, one reinforced by the Hawke government's leaving ministers a free hand within their portfolios. (Plummer, 1989, p. 31)

Allied to this possible explanation was the existence of a group of ministers/ministerial staff members and senior bureaucrats at the start of the epidemic who were either gay, or very supportive of the gay community. The role of personalities in shaping the policy response to HIV in Australia cannot be underestimated. The fact that gay or gay sympathetic individuals occupied key positions in government and the bureaucracy meant that Australia's response would incorporate the advice provided by members of the gay community. A fourth possible explanation for the involvement of gay community representatives is related to the anxieties and phobias of some politicians and bureaucrats. Could it be that they wished to be at 'arms' length' from the issue of HIV and distanced from those affected by the virus, namely gay men, IDUs, sex workers – and even distanced from illness and death?

Despite a 'maturing' of attitudes in relation to a number of social phenomena in Australia, homophobia and other similarly distasteful phobias continue to exist in Australia today:

Homophobia and phobias of people at risk of AIDS continually undermine our national AIDS response. It is a powerful manipulative tool
that has been shamelessly used with detrimental effects. (Plummer,
1989, p. 5)

Ross (1992) supports this view, referring to the continued use of the term
'innocent victims' to describe those people with medically acquired HIV. The
term has never been used by those organizations representing people with
haemophilia; rather 'it is regularly used by people (or their representatives)
who have been HIV infected by other transmission routes, or the media who
see the words as emotive and eye-catching' (Ross, 1992, p. 6).

The inclusion of community groups could also be the result of a deliberate
government policy to utilize 'health promotion' principles. Health promotion
principles may have been engaged to fight two foes: one was HIV; the other,
the dominant position of the medical profession in Australia. As Keenan and
van Reyk (1993, p. 2) observed: 'Debate in Australia about the broad direction
of health policy in HIV/AIDS has centred on the opposition of a traditional,
conservative approach to public health policy and practice, and a progressive
approach based on the principles of the Ottawa Charter'.

The significant effect of the use of health promotion principles to fight
HIV/AIDS has been a 'demedicalization' of policy in this field. The medical
community has repeatedly decried this development. Speaking at the 1988
National AIDS Conference in Hobart, a representative of the Australian Medical Association (AMA) commented that 'it has always been in the interest of
some groups to ensure that the AIDS epidemic remains primarily a political
issue not a public health issue' (Phillips, 1988, p. 640).

Phillips sought to remind his audience that AIDS is essentially an infectious disease and, as such, the medical profession has primary responsibility
for both prevention and management. The AMA's 1991 policy document on
AIDS reiterated this line, stating that AIDS 'is in essence a viral infection
spread mainly by contact with infected blood and genital secretions'; they
did, however, acknowledge that HIV has 'major social and moral implications' (AMA, 1991, p. 3). The AMA position is that HIV/AIDS should be
controlled using the 'usual principles of control of communicable disease'
(AMA, 1991, p. 3). The 1991 document further added that the AMA 'believes
that some of the advice the Australian Health Ministers have received from
government advisory bodies is contrary to sound public health principles'
(AMA, 1991, p. 3).

One of the most famous attacks on the health promotion approach to
HIV/AIDS came from the late Professor Fred Hollows in 1992 when he accused
the gay lobby of hijacking the national HIV/AIDS policy-making agenda. This
concept of a policy 'hijack' is not new in Australian health policy. Browning's
1987 article detailed the hostility caused by what was claimed to be the involvement of a 'host of "community" organisations' in health policy-making. Dwyer
(1989, p. 16) comments on the rationale behind such attacks, noting that 'I

suspect that when commentators deplore the clamour of too many competing interests in health and welfare policy debates, they are regretting that community voices have been added to those of other vested interests.'

Speaking at a conference in May 1992, Don Baxter, then Secretary of AFAO, put the AIDS 'hijack' controversy into a more realistic perspective:

> Underlying the current media storm is a deeper debate: whether 'control' of HIV/AIDS strategy should return to what are called the 'traditional public health' models, or whether the 'new public health' model, embodied in the Ottawa Charter principles, should continue to fashion our responses to the AIDS epidemic. (Baxter, 1992, p. 2)

Australian Federation of AIDS Organizations (AFAO)

The Australian Federation of AIDS Organizations is the peak umbrella organization for AIDS/HIV community organizations in Australia. Its constituent organizations include the state- and territory-based AIDS Councils, the National Association of People Living with HIV/AIDS, the Australian IV League and the Scarlet Alliance. The Haemophilia Foundation of Australia is not, and has never been, affiliated with AFAO.

Relationship with the 'Gay' Community

AFAO has made no attempt to disguise the fact that many of the people it represents are from the gay community. In 1991 AFAO adopted a charter on gay and lesbian issues which formally:

> recognises AFAO's special relationship with the gay and lesbian communities given the significant number of gay men with HIV/AIDS in Australia, the impact of the epidemic on this community, and the contribution of this community in response to AIDS/HIV. (Carr, 1991, p. 31)

In releasing the Charter, AFAO stated that it was 'an important step towards ensuring that gay men are actively involved in community-based AIDS organisations, and that AIDS organisations have a strong interaction with the gay and lesbian communities' (Carr, 1991, p. 31). The then President of AFAO, Bill Whittaker, commented on the visibility of gay men in the AIDS debate, noting:

There are many gay men involved in AIDS organisations, myself included. However, we are often constrained in speaking out as gay men because we wear 'other hats'. AIDS organisations need to adopt strategies to ensure that gay men do not become invisible in the debate about an epidemic which is most affecting them. (Carr, 1991, p. 31)

AFAO today receives representations from a wide range of non-AIDS gay and lesbian community groups. While not providing any financial support for such organizations, AFAO has on many occasions offered moral support. AFAO also actively lobbies on behalf of gay and lesbian community groups.

Relationship with the Medical Community

The relationship of AFAO with the medical community has not been an easy one, particularly its relationship with the AMA. Historically, the AMA has demonstrated specific homophobic and anti-community involvement tendencies – this was particularly evident during the presidency of Bruce Shepherd. The election of Brendan Nelson, a Tasmanian GP, as federal AMA president in 1993 heralded a new era for the AMA, especially in its relations with the wider community. For instance, the AMA and AFAO have since agreed to work jointly on initiatives or programmes 'which might be of mutual benefit to our two organisations and constituencies' (AFAO letter to AMA, 9 August 1993). The AMA has committed itself 'to be available to [AFAO] or your representatives to discuss initiatives for which you may seek our support or alternatively programmes upon which the AMA may be asked for public comment' (AMA letter to AFAO, 22 June 1993). In a speech to the National Press Club on 29 September 1993, Nelson stated that 'it is long past time to repeal the criminal code in Tasmania for homosexual activity' (Nelson, 1993, p. 11). While clearly stating that this was a personal view, the public nature of the statement clearly indicated an attempt to change more general perceptions of the Association.

The Position of Lesbians

It is obvious that gay men have benefited from their involvement in 'gay'-based community organizations. But what is the situation with lesbians? I have deliberately chosen to devote considerable attention to issues surrounding lesbians and AIDS for the following reasons. First, such a discussion highlights divisions within 'the gay community'. Second, lesbian sex is an area often avoided in the Australian HIV/AIDS literature. Thus, there exists considerable confusion and conjecture on this topic.

AFAO's Charter reaffirmed the role of gay people, both men and women,

in the AIDS debate; but in real life what is the situation? To classify any particular group as being at risk of HIV infection is inaccurate. Rather, it is risky
behaviours which place individuals at risk. While gay men account for the
vast majority of those infected in Australia, those infections result from individual behaviours and not from identification as gay men. This is not just a
debate about semantics; an understanding of the differences between sexual
identification and behaviours is essential in the development of appropriate
prevention strategies.

When the concept of risky behaviour is applied to lesbians, it appears
that lesbian sex offers minimal risk of viral transmission. There is no penile
penetration and provided that care is taken with sex during menstruation,
the risk of sharing bodily fluids is low. Infection through the use of sex toys
can be eliminated by following basic safer sex practices. 'Slip-ups', usually
associated with penile sex without condoms, perhaps while under the influence of drugs, are far less likely to occur in lesbian sex than in male-to-
female, or male-to-male sex.

When Whittaker (AFAO, 1991/92) spoke about the visibility of gay men
in the AIDS debate, he did not include the visibility of lesbians. Since the
emergence of the 'gay plague', lesbians have been particularly supportive of
gay men affected by the virus. They have provided financial and moral support;
perhaps more importantly, they have provided substantial support in terms of
personal care for those gay men affected by AIDS. This level of support is somewhat surprising given the history of gay male/lesbian relations in the past two
decades. Ever since the emergence of the gay liberation movement in the 1960s,
there has been a simmering animosity in Australia between 'poofters' and 'dykes'.
The two groups rarely agreed on political strategies – which is hardly surprising
given that it has never been illegal for two women to have sex together. Laws
prohibiting homosexual acts only applied to men. Thus, it was men only who
required law reform to protect their private consenting sexual practices. But
gay liberation developed in tandem with the feminist movement. Consequently
there emerged a commonality of purpose between the feminist movement
and the lesbian branch of gay liberation: men were perceived as the common
enemy, regardless of their sexual preference. The 'phallus' and the 'act of
penetration' emerged as the barricades between gay men and lesbians.

It was not until the mid-1980s that the two groups achieved some degree of accommodation between their different positions. Several factors may
account for this. First, with the emergence of AIDS, politically active gay men
diverted their efforts to that cause. This gave lesbians greater scope for political participation. A second factor may have been the decriminalization of
homosexuality in New South Wales, which resulted in gay men and lesbians
having equal footing before the law. Another factor undoubtedly influencing
the breakdown in animosity between the two groups has been the level of
political maturity which the gay liberation movement had achieved. The 'Gay
Lib' of the 1970s was dead: the 1980s was the decade of 'homosexual law
reform'. 'Inclusion' became the new catch-phrase.

Lesbians have noted that 'the AIDS crisis has given the gay male community a voice, but lesbian sexuality and lesbian lifestyles are as invisible to the general community as ever' (Drake, 1992, p. 23). Concluding that 'AIDS has become a vehicle for advancing a new vision of sexuality for all people', Drake claims that 'lesbians have a lot to benefit from this movement to broaden the community's view of human sexuality and all its complexities' (1992, p. 23). Drake further notes that because of the AIDS crisis, homosexuality has been made more visible to the general community – male homosexuality that is. Gay males are more visible than ever, while lesbians remain 'invisible'. 'For some lesbians, this invisibility is stifling and becomes more so as gay male sexuality receives increasing publicity' (Drake, 1992, p. 23). She even suggests that some lesbians have responded to the AIDS crisis, and particularly its concentration on gay males, by 'actively "piggy-backing" lesbian visibility on the AIDS issue' (1992, p. 23), thus leading to criticism that the lesbian community has, to a degree, hijacked the AIDS debate.

People Living with HIV/AIDS (PLWHAs)

The notion of a specific HIV/AIDS community implies that *all* individuals and organizations working in the HIV/AIDS field must remain focused on the prevention of new infections and the care of those already infected. In an address to the 1994 *HIV, AIDS and Society Conference* held at Macquarie University, Andrew Morgan, representing PLWHAs, noted that some sections of the broader 'community' were not maintaining that focus. While acknowledging the important work carried out by social researchers, Morgan criticized that same group for being preoccupied with research on transmission of the virus and neglecting the impact of infection on those living with and dying from HIV.

Within the AIDS community (using the broad definition offered earlier by Ariss) there exists a number of policy agendas – perhaps as many as the number of organizations working in this field. This is quite reasonable given the multifaceted nature of the issues relating to HIV. Yet there exists an undercurrent of concern – and in some cases exasperation – that the situation of HIV-positive people, particularly those with serious illness, is being ignored by many in the AIDS community. In some cases this undercurrent of concern has developed into outright conflict: for instance, ACT UP developed out of – and is sustained by – the fact that many HIV-positive people believe that existing AIDS CBOs fail to represent their situation.

In Australia, many PLWHA groups have deliberately not affiliated with existing AIDS councils or AFAO. Individual PLWHAs are now also publicly speaking out about lack of representation; for many such individuals this process is extremely difficult. For many, 'coming out' as a gay man is difficult enough, 'coming out' as an HIV-positive person can be even more confronting; 'coming out' as an HIV-positive gay man who is critical of the very organizations designed to represent their case is seen by some as being the ultimate betrayal. Yet, increasingly, more HIV-positive people are doing so. In a letter to the Federal Minister for Health dated 16 October 1993, Martyn Goddard (a journalist and AIDS activist) stated:

> In more than a decade of AIDS, there has still been no substantial campaign directed at HIV positive gay men. It's been too politically difficult: there has been too much concern that such a campaign could lead to discrimination and to rejection by its target group. There are real difficulties that need to be overcome, but they are not insuperable. This matter needs to come out of the too-hard basket. (Joyce, 1991, p. 33)

In 1991 an AFAO Committee held a workshop entitled 'Taking on board the needs of HIV infected people – the challenge for AFAO member organisations', during which three main areas of need were identified. These included PLWHA representation on boards of management and workplace plans; the training of staff and volunteers; and measures to ensure access to programmes and projects. Following the workshop, AFAO stated that they will 'develop a plan to oversee skills-sharing, promote forward planning and develop a review mechanism for the changing and varying needs of HIV infected people' (Carr, 1991, p. 33). However, in 1996, PLWHAs continue to call for their needs to be adequately addressed.

ACT UP

The AIDS Coalition to Unleash Power (ACT UP) developed out of dissatisfaction with the existing government and community-based organizations. A substantial component of ACT UP's activities have been associated with gaining easier and quicker access to drug treatments for people with HIV. ACT UP/Canberra, for example, were 'horrified' with various aspects of the 1991 Baume report on the provision of therapeutic drugs. They clearly felt not only under-represented, but also misrepresented by AFAO on this issue, concluding:

> Many of us have close ties to organisations which constitute AFAO and do not believe that adequate consultation has occurred regarding the previously jointly held position. The Government view AFAO as 'representing' many of us who do not feel well represented by your present stand. (ACT UP/Canberra letter to AFAO, 27 August 1991)

The same story of discontent with AFAO by members of ACT UP is demonstrated in correspondence from other chapters of the organization. Tony Westmore, on behalf of ACT UP/Sydney, wrote to AFAO on 20 June 1991 about the availability of therapeutic goods (drugs) for people with HIV/AIDS. At the time ACT UP was involved in an extensive campaign on this issue. In relation to the concept of an 'AIDS partnership' the letter stated:

> This partnership, comprised of various individuals and organisations including AFAO, has been described as fragile. We hope so. This partnership is nothing of the sort. It is a conspiracy of silence, which, in combination with several other factors, is killing people at the rate of five per week.

The letter continued:

> The 'AIDS movement' in Australia in June 1991 is leaderless, decisionless and about to be royally screwed. You are responsible for this situation also. Directly. Huge amounts of 'work' and minimal resources do not justify the absolute fuck-up AFAO has made of the drug approval/availability issue.

The letter concluded on a slightly more conciliatory note:

> Sadly, a degree of acrimony between our organisations is now evident. We will do what we can to improve relations as opportunities arise to do so. (ACT UP/Sydney letter to AFAO, 20 June 1991)

AFAO's relations with other chapters of ACT UP have not been necessarily negative. The Melbourne chapter, for instance, appreciated a positive association with AFAO. In July 1991 they wrote to AFAO 'petitioning' support from AFAO and its member organizations about education campaigns stressing the use of water-based lubricants with condoms. In concluding their letter they requested that:

> AFAO lobby ANCA, and the Commonwealth Department of Community Services and Health to take up this issue through their National Media Campaign, and all the other relevant material produced by them. (ACT UP/Melbourne to AFAO 24 July 1991)

The Future of Community-based Organizations (CBOs)

Alford (1977, p. 220) notes that individuals who have been involved in community participation in health are 'likely to become discouraged and leave, or will be co-opted into one of the established health organisations'. Such developments can be observed in AIDS CBOs in Australia.

'Burnout' among the volunteer sector of AIDS organizations is common in Australia. There are also a number of prominent CBO workers who have been engaged professionally with AIDS organizations who have come from, and moved on to, other senior positions, principally within the bureaucracy, international organizations and ministerial offices. The bureaucratization and professionalization of AIDS CBOs have been a major concern for members of such organizations.

It is clear that AIDS councils have been successful in community building, thus promoting a sense of gay community identity. However, the future role for AIDS councils seems somewhat unclear. The impact of HIV on the community is changing direction: prevention and education have been responsible for the decrease in new infection rates: because of the long lead time in progression from infection to the onset of AIDS, those who were infected in the early to mid-1980s are now becoming sick.

Altman (1993, p. 8) claims that many community-based organizations now reflect the dominant structures of the existing health bureaucracy and that AIDS councils have become more like 'mini-health departments'. Professionals, rather than community representatives, have come to control the policy processes, which is seen in some quarters as a challenge to the *raison d'être* for many of these organizations. The appointment of highly skilled professionals to AIDS councils has placed internal strains on these organizations between members/volunteers and staff (Altman, 1990, p. 17). This is true of all voluntary organizations, but is possibly felt more strongly in the AIDS area where psychological investments in the issue are so great. AIDS organizations increasingly have to cope with illness and death among key volunteers and staff, which creates extraordinary stress for the organizations (Altman, 1990, p. 17).

Dowsett (1992, p. 6) suggests that the incorporation of community groups into mainstream policy processes is not unique to the AIDS field, reflecting that through the bureaucratization of Australian AIDS CBOs, 'there appears to be a growing danger that gay communities might follow one trajectory in modern feminism of producing, for the few, certain career paths, while relegating the rest to a "minority" status *cul de sac* in post-industrial pluralism'.

Members of the gay community have strenuously resisted attempts to dehomosexualize AIDS community-based organizations. Such organizations have been threatened on two fronts: first, through a process of professionalization and, second, through attempts to broaden the categories of those said to be at risk (Carr, 1989, pp. 5–6). At times, particularly during the 'Grim Reaper' period, prevention campaigns have been aimed at a wide cross-section of the Australian community. The fact remains, however, that even in 1996 gay men still account for well over 85 per cent of all cases of HIV infection. Thus, the *raison d'être* for AIDS organizations which represent specific groups remains the same as it did in the early days of the epidemic.

Conclusions

The Australian response to HIV/AIDS can be regarded as 'exceptional' in several respects. First, the response to date departs from policy-making norms because it actively encourages the participation of affected communities. Through this process, groups in society previously considered marginalized have been considerably empowered. The response can also be regarded as exceptional because state and territory governments, with which the constitutional responsibility for all health matters rests, have allowed the Commonwealth to take the lead in HIV/AIDS policy development. This situation is unusual in the Australian context as states' rights are usually strongly protected by the states and territories. Another departure from the Australian norm is the fact that HIV/AIDS policy has enjoyed a high degree of bipartisan support among the major political parties.

In March 1996 a new national government was elected with a policy of devolving responsibilities back to the states and territories, as well as an overall policy of reducing government activities and spending. Since the election, HIV/AIDS community-based organizations have expressed concern about the future directions of the existing partnership. The election coincided with planning for the Third National HIV/AIDS Strategy.

Policies of the new government in relation to all policy areas, including HIV/AIDS, were not known at the time of writing: the new government has announced that future policy directions would be revealed in the context of the annual budget due to be handed down in August 1996. Several general aspects of future directions in HIV/AIDS policy are, however, clear. The process of mainstreaming begun during the term of the previous government will continue. The new Health Minister, Michael Woolridge, has also announced that there will be a Third National Strategy and that the process of consultation with affected communities will continue under the new government. The Australian HIV/AIDS communities are yet to be convinced that future directions in policy will build on the investments of the past.

References

ACT UP (1991) letter to AFAO, 27 August.
AFAO ARCHIVES:
    AFAO Archive 4.2.1.
    ACT UP/Sydney letter to AFAO, 20 June 1991.
    ACT UP/Melbourne letter to AFAO, 24 July 1991.
    ACT UP/Canberra letter to AFAO, 27 August 1991.

AFAO (1991/92) *National AIDS Bulletin,* 5, 1, p. 31.

AMA letter to AFAO, 22 June 1993.

AFAO letter to AMA, 9 August 1993.

ALFORD, R.R. (1977) *Health Care Politics,* Chicago: The University of Chicago Press.

ALTMAN, D. (1990) 'Community-based organisations and the future', *National AIDS Bulletin,* 4, 1, pp. 16–18.

ALTMAN, D. (1993) 'Expertise, legitimacy and the centrality of community', in P. AGGLETON, P. DAVIES and G. HART (Eds) *AIDS: Facing the Second Decade,* London: Falmer Press.

ARON, P. (1991) 'An expanded role for community organisations', in N.F. MACKENZIE (Ed.) *The AIDS Reader: Social, Political, Ethical Issues,* New York: Meridian.

AUSTRALIAN MEDICAL ASSOCIATION (1991) *Policy on HIV/AIDS,* Canberra: Australian Medical Association.

CARR, A. (1989) 'Why we have AIDS Councils', *National AIDS Bulletin,* 3, 2, pp. 5–6.

CARR, A. (1991) 'The HIV epidemic: the next ten years', *National AIDS Bulletin,* 5, 6, pp. 9–13.

CARR, A. (1992) 'When we were very young: the early years of the HIV/AIDS epidemic in Victoria', *National AIDS Bulletin,* 6, 6, pp. 15–17.

CROFTS, N. (1992) 'Patterns of infection', in E. TIMEWELL, V. MINCHINIELLO and D. PLUMMER (Eds) *AIDS in Australia,* Sydney: Prentice Hall.

DOWSETT, G. (1992) 'Practising desire: homosexual sex in the era of AIDS', unpublished PhD Thesis, Sydney: Macquarie University.

DAVIS, G., WANNA, J., WARHURST, J. and WELLER, P. (Eds) (1988) *Public Policy in Australia,* Boston: Allen & Unwin.

DRAKE, M. (1992) 'Lesbian visibility at what price?', *National AIDS Bulletin,* 6, 1, pp. 23–4.

DWYER, J. (1989) 'The politics of participation', in M. MILLER and R. WALKER (Eds) *Health Promotion: The Community Health Approach,* papers from the 2nd Conference of the Australian Community Health Association, Sydney: Australian Community Health Association.

GRAY, G. (1987) 'Health policy in two federations', unpublished PhD Thesis, Canberra: Australian National University.

HOWE, B. (1992) 'Keynote Address' paper given at the *AIDS: Have we got it right?* Conference, Sydney, May.

JORDAN, A.G. (1981) 'Iron triangles, woolly corporatism and elastic nets: images of the policy process', *Journal of Public Policy,* 1, 1, pp. 95–123.

JOYCE, L. (1991) 'AFAO committee meeting', *National AIDS Bulletin,* 5, 4, p. 33.

KEENAN, T. and VAN REYK, P. (1993) 'Lobbying for change: the Australian experience of HIV/AIDS', paper given at the *HIV/AIDS Law, Policy and Directions Conference,* Melbourne, October.

NELSON, B. (1993) Speech at the National Press Club, 22 June.

PHILLIPS, B. (1988) 'The role of the Australian Medical Association', paper given at the *Hobart National AIDS Conference.*

PLUMMER, D. (1989) 'Homophobia: the fear of AIDS prevention?', *National AIDS Bulletin,* 3, 5, p. 4.

PLUMMER, K. (1988) 'The culture of AIDS, the politics of AIDS, worlds apart', in P. AGGLETON and H. HOMANS (Eds) *Social Aspects of AIDS*, Lewes: Falmer Press.

PLWHA (1994) *1994 Annual Conference Prospectus.*

PROSS, A.P. (1986) *Group Politics and Public Policy*, Oxford: Oxford University Press.

ROSS, J. (1992) Unpublished paper given at the *AIDS: Have we got it right?* Conference, Sydney, May.

VAN REYK, P. (1990) (Ed.) *The Frontline View of the National HIV/AIDS Strategy: Selected Papers from the 4th National Conference on HIV/AIDS, 4 August 1990 Canberra*, Canberra: ACON.

WATSON, C. (1993) 'The nature of HIV/AIDS', paper given at the *HIV/AIDS Law, Policy and Directions Conference*, Melbourne, October.

Chapter 5

Constraints in the Development of Sexual Health Alliances

Roger Ingham, Emily Jaramazović and Diane Stevens

In England (as elsewhere), it is well documented (for example, Allen, 1987; Hutton, 1992; Thomson and Scott, 1992; Woodcock, Stenner and Ingham, 1992; Evans, Ingham and Roots, 1994; NFER, 1994) that there are limitations on what schools can achieve in terms of sex education. Among the various problems are the lack of adequate training for teachers, the difficulties of dealing with large classes, a tendency to concentrate too much on the biological aspects of reproduction, the difficulties of dealing with 'sensitive issues' through embarrassment and/or fears of possible parental reaction, the pressures on curriculum time as a result of the National Curriculum and league tables of examination results,[1] and so on. Recent changes to the Education Act, including the right of young people to withdraw (or be withdrawn by their parents) from sex-education classes and the ambiguity about the legal position of teachers giving advice, have further added to the problems associated with placing too much faith in school-based sex-education programmes.

For these and other reasons, alternative opportunities for sex and sexuality education need to be developed. Even if highly effective school-based programmes were to be introduced in the near future, it would take some years for their benefits to take effect. Community-based programmes are therefore needed to complement and support school-based programmes and to provide for all those who need them and who are not in full-time education. Various possibilities exist and it is important to explore their potential if *The Health of the Nation* targets on sexual health are to be achieved.[2]

In the same way, however, that there are changing circumstances in schools, so there are in the various alternative potential community settings for the delivery of sex education. Current and future changes in the health service are likely to have an impact on the opportunities to plan and implement effective initiatives.

The study reported here[3] involved the selection of eight sites in England, with a mix of urban and rural, geographical spread, and other indices. In each site, between ten and twelve detailed interviews were conducted with staff from a range of agencies, including health, education, social services, youth service and voluntary organizations. Initial contact was made through the appropriate District HIV/AIDS Prevention Coordinators (DHPCs), who suggested the key players in each site. But to avoid the possibility of their suggesting only people with whom they had good relations, other avenues were also used to obtain suitable participants. In general, the DHPCs were extremely helpful in making local arrangements, despite this being yet another study from which they might not directly benefit!

For each site, copies of relevant publications were obtained in advance, including the AIDS (Control) Act reports,[4] sexual health strategy documents, purchasing plans, the Director of Public Health's Annual Reports and needs' assessments conducted. The standard protocol of the interviews covered (1) past and present initiatives in the field of sexual health; (2) the nature of, and problems, with alliances; (3) the availability of sexual health services and support, including specially targeted provision; (4) the nature of the purchaser-provider relationships, contracts and the use of quality measures; (5) the reactions of local media and politicians to sexual health initiatives; (6) future plans and priorities in the field of sexual health, together with the likely effects of the removal of ring-fenced prevention money; and (7) the potential barriers to the fruition of the perceived priorities. The majority of respondents had plenty to say on all these areas and in most cases were extremely honest and forthcoming (as far as we could tell). Respondents were assured of anonymity and confidentiality and all interviews were tape-recorded and transcribed verbatim.

Obviously, there is a great deal of interesting material in these transcripts. For the purpose of this chapter, however, we concentrate on the area of sexual health alliances. Before we outline some of the data gathered, it is worth reminding ourselves what is meant by the term 'alliances'. *The Health of the Nation Key Area Handbook on HIV/AIDS and Sexual Health* (Department of Health, 1993, pp. 14–15) provides a useful outline:

> Improving and promoting sexual health is not the sole responsibility of the NHS. *The Health of the Nation* makes it clear that the key objectives cannot be achieved without involving other agencies and organisations which may have differing but complementary roles to play. These include Local Authorities, other statutory and non-statutory organisations, community services and voluntary groups. Healthy alliances offer imaginative and flexible approaches to local inter-agency co-operation, working across boundaries with the objective of improving the health of the population, as well as increasing collaboration between the different agencies and within the NHS. Alliances can: overcome barriers . . . create synergy . . . avoid unnecessary duplication . . . act as a catalyst . . . and are participative.

An 'ideal' model might involve a fully developed action plan, based on detailed needs' assessments, with each agency providing appropriate services and support reflecting their own expertise and interests, with this total community provision being accessible by all people as and when required.

Key Findings

Throughout the analysis that follows, our overall focus is on what we perceived to be constraints in the development of healthy alliances in the field of sexual health. Not surprisingly, the level and range of community-based activities varied quite considerably between sites, with a rather wider range of activities and target groups in the urban than the rural sites (although the small sample size makes it difficult to make too much of this tendency). All sites contained highly motivated and committed groups of people, and their dedication, in most cases, could not be doubted. If any of the comments that follow appear somewhat critical, they are certainly not intended to apply to any particular individuals. As we hope will become clear, the structural changes which were being introduced into the health and other services, together with uncertainty over future funding arrangements, contributed to a rather uncoordinated and sometimes chaotic picture. Indeed, that there are so many initiatives being undertaken under such circumstances is, in itself, an indication of hope.

Variations in Definitions of Sexual Health and Priorities

The first area concerns definitional aspects of sexual health. Not surprisingly, there was quite a wide range of priorities among the respondents – presumably, alliances will work more effectively in cases where there is general agreement about the aims of service provision and intended outcomes.

In most sites, the White Paper had had the effect of shifting the emphasis of activities away from specific HIV/AIDS initiatives towards a more general concept of sexual health. Many respondents mentioned that they, and/or their managers, felt 'more comfortable' with this wider definition, either at a personal level, or because it made it easier to justify claims for resources from fund-holders. As we shall mention later, this wider definition permitted initiatives to be aimed at 'young people' in general (of which there are many) rather than other groups in the community whose prevalence is less clear.

· This shift did, however, lead to resentment in some sites: those who had been working for some time in targeted outreach activities with particular groups felt their efforts were being undermined and marginalized. This sometimes worked the other way as well: a degree of resentment was mentioned by some respondents that the particular priorities of those in control of funding led to too many resources going to minority group interests. The tensions raised by this apparent shift from HIV/AIDS prevention approaches (which tended to target gay men, drug users and sex-workers) towards wider sexual health issues (with an emphasis on young people in general) were not always conducive to the aim of working together in a trusting and collaborative atmosphere.

In addition to this overall shift in emphasis there were, not surprisingly, a wide range of other definitions of sexual health mentioned by respondents. In general, those nearer to the decision-making process were concerned with the government's *Health of the Nation* targets, whereas those working more directly with the community (such as outreach workers, youth services and voluntary organizations) tended to have less clearly defined objectives. Thus, for example, youth club leaders reported being encouraged to:

> create open situations where children [*sic*] have the opportunity to discuss their own personal feelings and values about unwanted pregnancy, underage sex and termination of pregnancy in a safe environment before they are in a position of having to make a decision.

An outreach worker mentioned that:

> I aim to access the disadvantaged and young people to improve choices or empower them to make informed choices about their sexual health . . . ultimately to ensure that they can discuss sex and practise safer sex.

A street-based peer education project was designed to:

> make contact with young people who are unlikely to be in contact with existing services and build relationships with them, empowering them to make informed choices about their bodies, their relationships and their lives.

A number of others referred to the importance of 'self-esteem', one youth worker suggesting that 'If you feel good about yourself you will not put yourself under threat.' Other priorities mentioned included the perceived need to challenge many of the attitudes of those in positions of authority, be they members of health authorities and commissions, school governors or local politicians. These respondents argued that specific targeted interventions would cease once ringfenced money no longer existed, and that major changes in attitude would be needed in many areas of society. Such changes would include attention being paid to the discrimination and stigmatization of certain groups, challenging the 'ingrained attitudes' of many that talking about sex encourages young people to do it and challenging many myths which exist in relation to sexual conduct. All respondents had some clear ideas about the future needs in their localities, and these were generally pretty comprehensive 'wish-lists'. However, there was a general sense of pessimism about the likelihood of these being taken forward, with both financial and attitudinal reasons being cited.

When discussing alliances, many respondents pointed to the difficulties of working harmoniously together when the different parties involved had such varied agendas. Although many of the specific aims of individual respondents, some of which are cited above, could be regarded as essential prerequisites for achieving the more objective targets of the funders, little effort appears to have been made in any of the sites to work through this process of integration. There were various reasons for this, some of which are mentioned below, but a lack of mutual understanding of what each other was trying to achieve was a major one. A vivid example was provided by the respondent (echoing others) who reported:

> I've been requested by fellow managers to take down posters with condoms on them because it made them feel physically sick, and they will say so at senior meetings of managers; they are not embarrassed to say so, in fact they feel quite noble.

We have carried out some detailed discourse analyses[5] of the ways in which respondents working in different agencies talked about their views of sexual health and associated issues; presumably, alliances will work more effectively where there is some evidence of common discursive approaches to the whole area.

A Case Study

To take one complete site as an illustration, many respondents believed that if certain misunderstandings were cleared up between the key agencies involved in education in community settings, alliances will form, prosper and dovetail to meet the same ends. However, discourse analysis of the transcripts of interviews conducted in this site reveals that rather than being involved in the same endeavour, working towards common goals for broadly similar reasons, there are marked differences in how the key players conceptualize sexual behaviour, sex education and desired outcomes. In many ways, these key players are speaking different languages, with alliances providing little in the way of translation.

For example, the purchasers saw the greatest need as targeting young women because of the high teenage pregnancy rate. Levels of service provision were of major concern, with education seen as being of secondary importance. Their view was that one's sexual health is one's own responsibility: 'At the end of the day it is your choice or my choice what you do with your life and whether you do or you do not have a sexually transmitted disease.' For them, providing accessible clinics is the key to reducing teenage pregnancy rates. They were not so much concerned with what people do, but with them not becoming pregnant, or if they do, having access to termination services. Family planning clinic clientèle are mainly female, and extra resources are given to geographical areas of high pregnancy rates. The underlying assumption was that if a young female client is sexually active, she will not stop having sex, but if she comes in for advice and is still a virgin, you should send her away to think about it.

Service providers, on the other hand, conceptualized the problem rather differently, depending on their particular focus. The DHPC role is seen more in the wider context of sexual health, as issues such as teenage pregnancy all stem from unsafe sex. Occasionally, funding had to be liberated, rather than focusing on the actual needs of the groups who need financial support, by playing to heterosexual fears of HIV infection; for example, by revealing that HIV-positive drug users were having heterosexual sex with women in the area.

Many health service personnel felt that the *Health of the Nation* targets would not be met until there were drastic changes within the education service. The Education Department employs a specialist adviser with a partial remit to get sexual health education on people's agenda. The postholder saw the main functions of this role to protect teachers from criticism of the way they provide sex education, and to promote the importance of morality in sex education. Community education work was also targeting young women within a feminist perspective, based round notions of confidence, self-defense, esteem-raising and empowerment.

Gay community development work funded by the social services in the district aimed to reduce HIV infection by increasing choices around safer sex. Although reasonably well-funded, the project workers were cynical of the value placed on their efforts, believing there is a hidden agenda, and there is no real interest in gay issues, just fears concerning married closet homosexuals: 'poor married men might spread the plague to their nice little heterosexual wives'. Generally, problems were reported in relation to making others accept the worth of their endeavour:

There is a low expectation of professionalism of projects like this . . . whenever you meet new professionals like GPs they are expecting you to be a kind of gay volunteer nobody and when you say 'I am employed by social services' they are really quite surprised, it is quite good actually because they are immediately impressed.

Voluntary organizations, for example the Youth Council, expressed similar concerns. 'If you do work on a shoestring budget you're not taken seriously, and other agencies expect youth workers to put in additional voluntary work.' The various conceptualizations of sexual behaviour and sex education geared towards meeting the targets set in the *Health of the Nation* can be understood with reference to the following discursive themes:

Power, Control and Agenda-Setting

Health professionals generally had adequate funding to employ full-time workers, and were more often represented on formal alliances around policy issues than were those working in education, with those working at grass-roots level, particularly in gay community-development work, being hardly represented at all. Mainstream service providers had a top–down approach to needs' assessment, whereas voluntary agencies placed greater emphasis on the needs of the groups they serve. While in this district there was a commitment from many sectors to peer education, it was woefully underfunded and the workers were aware of the lack of professionalism credited to them.

Female Heterosexuality and Male Homosexuality as Negative Forces

When targeting groups, most organizations focused on young people, mainly women, as the major problem was thought to be unwanted teenage pregnancies. However, a focus on pregnancy and young women obscured the dyadic nature of sexual behaviour and fostered an impression of negative female sexuality. Similarly, community development focused exclusively on gay men, making the issue problem-centred (AIDS, STDs) rather than sexuality-centred. Pregnant teenagers had been targeted even though many health professionals, including service purchasers, acknowledged that the root of the problem lay elsewhere; while they recognized unwanted pregnancies and sexually transmitted diseases as wider social issues, they concentrated their efforts on small-scale single-agency solutions.

Empowerment Versus Damage Limitation

Most health and mainstream educational workers conceptualized sex education as a form of damage limitation rather than seeing the benefits of a sexual education in its own right. Community development workers, however, with their focus on empowerment, celebrated sexuality in its entirety, not just focusing on problematic outcomes.

Needs Assessments and Evaluation

The varying agendas of different agencies also affected the nature of the needs' assessment process, as well as the seriousness with which it was taken. Few local profiles had been produced in the way envisaged by the government's *Key Area Handbook*, and little attention appeared to be paid to national or international research findings. Some sites had conducted questionnaire studies in schools to assess knowledge and risk behaviours, while others relied on general notions of national priorities or 'common sense'.

Many provider respondents felt alienated from the needs' assessment and prioritization process, feeling that priorities were imposed from above and that their local knowledge was not properly valued and respected. The (then) upcoming regional mergers were seen as a threat to locally based needs' assessments,[6] it was assumed that fewer staff would be required to cover much larger geographical areas and that sensitivity to local issues would be lost as a result. The emphasis on young people in general led to the assumption that more drop-in clinics were required. Whereas this is a highly defensible policy, there was little evidence of there being any careful analysis of where these were most needed.

A few sites mentioned what might be termed 'negative needs' assessment'. In these cases, decisions had been taken by those in authority that specialized provision for, for example, gay men was not required since (in their view) the area did not have any. This had lead to some resentment in several sites where clients from neighbouring districts were being catered for, but no financial help was being received from their authorities.

In the absence of clearly articulated needs' assessments, it was not surprising that evaluation was reported to be rather *ad hoc* and somewhat sparse. Clinics tended to rely on client throughput as a major measure of success, although in these cases little attention was paid to what might be called the 'value-added' nature of these contacts. In other words, although numbers were recorded, no attention was given to the specific needs of the particular clients attending, nor the time required to support them adequately. Similarly, there was a feeling that too much emphasis was placed on user-satisfaction surveys. Whereas these were regarded as important in themselves, many respondents argued that it would actually be more useful to conduct non-user surveys, in order more fully to understand the barriers which prevented some people from using the services available.

Many respondents working closer to the community, and with wider aims than simple quantification, reported their frustrations at the difficulties they faced in the area of evaluation. For example, those who aimed to improve 'self-esteem' or 'choices' reported problems of convincing those in authority that improvements were occurring, and commented on the apparent reluctance of the 'decision-makers' to accept qualitative data as providing appropriate evidence of success. The vast majority of respondents reported that they would like to receive a great deal more support in the whole area of needs' assessment and evaluation.

Impact of Changes in the Health Service

Perhaps the greatest barrier to the formation of healthy alliances was the impact of the changes in the health service (and, to some extent, in social services), including mergers, the introduction of the purchaser-provider model[7] and other factors which created uncertainties. Although quite a few respondents reported that, in principle, the notion of being more accountable and having clearer objectives was, in itself, not a bad thing, the effects of the changing climate were generally very negative. There were a number of ways in which the effects were experienced.

Mergers

At the time of the study, many district health authorities were in the process of merging with family health service authorities to become commissions, and regions were beginning to be combined in preparation for their eventual demise. This created a sense of uncertainty and fear among many respondents who, not unnaturally, did not feel inclined to enter into close alliances with others when they were not sure if they, or their post, would still be there in a few months' time. It was generally assumed that mergers would lead to fewer posts and that respondents' own jobs were at risk. In this context, others carrying out similar duties in a neighbouring district or region were seen as potential rivals for future posts. The effort needed to set up and actively foster alliances was not thought to be worthwhile with such uncertain futures.

This climate of uncertainty also led to rapid staff turnover and some respondents pointed to the frustrations of having made efforts to establish relationships with other workers, only to find that they later departed for other posts. A further impact of rapid staff turnover was the relatively long time that posts were left vacant and, in some cases, other staff in the agency were unable to stand in for the person who had left. Some potentially exciting joint initiatives had simply ceased to continue under these circumstances.

A further impact of mergers was that many respondents felt that the decision-making processes were being further and further removed from the work at ground level, and that financial considerations were playing an increasing role in what was and what was not to be funded. This led to increasing feelings of being undervalued, especially among those working with marginalized sectors of the community.

Purchaser-provider Model

At the time of the study, the purchaser-provider model was in its very early stages of implementation, so it is perhaps not surprising that there was a great deal of confusion among many of the respondents. Indeed, some respondents to whom we spoke did not know on which side of the divide they were and several others reported that they spent half the week being purchasers and the other half being service providers.

In the majority of cases, existing arrangements had been continued, with existing providers being asked to continue their work. However, this was recognized as a short-term policy and that more detailed negotiations would be needed once the system had settled down. Fears were expressed about the nature of the contracts which would eventually be needed, and the risk of a shift towards purely quantitative means of assessing service provision. For those working to the wider aims mentioned above, this posed a serious challenge, since simple headcounts did not, in their view, provide an adequate measure of the quality of their provision.

This continuation of the current arrangements meant that, in practice, one of the government's aims in introducing the purchaser-provider model – to increase efficiency through encouraging competition – was not occurring. In most sites, there was only one possible provider for a particular service, so a monopoly situation effectively existed. However, the changed nature of the relationship had led to an increase in the level of paperwork required (what the economists term 'transactions costs') and this was resented by many respondents. Some organizations – especially in the voluntary sector – were simply not equipped to change their working practices so drastically and they felt that other work suffered as a result.

Related to this issue was a strong feeling among many voluntary organizations that the details in their contracts were stricter than those being established with other parts of the health service (many of the health service arrangements constituted only minor parts of much larger block contracts placed with a Trust). This differential treatment was perceived by many voluntary organizations to indicate a lack of trust and closer control regarding their activities. However, one purchaser defended this position by emphasizing that they were attempting to encourage and steer the local voluntary organizations through being more explicit about the expectations and support required.

Although there was little evidence, if any, of *actual* competitive tendering between agencies, many respondents were aware of the *potential* of the changing environment. These perceptions had some negative effects on the formation of healthy alliances. For example, many respondents from agencies who all believed that they could provide a particular service reported that they were unwilling to share their plans with potential competitors. This was particularly noticeable, for example, in the overlapping interests of family planning staff, school nurses, general practice staff (with the shift to GP fund-holders) and others who felt that they could provide sexual health services for young people, and some health promotion staff felt threatened by the increasing interest in sexual health shown by school nurses and others. As one respondent, discussing her contributions to the local sexual health forum, put it: 'For example, I would tell them what I'm doing, but only if it benefits us to do so.' She reported that 'In the old NHS we were part of a team – now people are fearful of losing their jobs or something and they want to hold on to it.'

Another said:

> If they are doing my job, then I am going to lose mine; you need to keep your boundaries clear, sort out which bits belong to who. With this market now you have to fight for money, for your job or the things you are interested in. You have to do that in a selfish way.

Other reported impacts of the shift towards the purchaser-provider model were shorter time horizons, faster staff turnover and a general increase in uncertainty. None of these was reported to be conducive to closer working alliances with other agencies.

Impact of Local Management of Schools

As well as substantial changes in the health services, changes in the education sector were also reported to be having an impact on the creation of multisectoral healthy alliances. These changes can be summarized as shifting the bulk of resources away from centralized education authority control down to the level of individual schools, leading to fewer staff being employed directly by the old authorities. These shifts, in addition to the removal of special temporary funding for health education initiatives, led to many of the sex education advisory staff losing their posts. In some cases these staff had been taken over by the local health authority or commission, whereas in other cases they had simply moved away from the area. This reduced the potential for close working relationships at a local level between health and education, although, as some of our respondents remarked, this simply reflects the national situation whereby the health and education sectors seem to have problems working together.

Some respondents pointed to the serious difficulties faced in liaising appropriately with the education sector, with schools having much more autonomy about the extent to which they take sexual health seriously. The joint planning of local provision was reported as being problematic when different schools in the area had varied levels of commitment; in some cases, schools' policies in this area were determined more by moral objections (by governors and staff) and/or the threat of the removal of students, than by needs' assessments or by playing their part in an integrated community approach. As one teacher of personal, social and health education put it: 'The image of the school is important – we are competing – every youngster who comes into our school is carrying money with them . . . you lose ten students, you lose £10 000: half a teacher.'

Personal Issues

One aim of healthy alliances is for agencies to work closely together to provide a comprehensive service. The global impression we received was that, in practice, personal factors as opposed to what might be called agency-level factors, affected whether or not alliances were successful. Obviously, personal likes and dislikes were expressed by the respondents and these appeared to play a large part in determining the willingness of people to work closely with others. In discussing local HIV and sexual health forums and alliances, many respondents commented on the great importance of being able to trust particular others in the group – although this may be inevitable in many settings, it did suggest to us that, where good alliances do appear to exist, they do so on a flimsy base. Should certain key individuals leave or move on to other posts, the momentum and impetus of jointly planned initiatives might well be lost. It was not always clear to us that there were firm agency commitments to the area which would survive the loss of key staff.

Related to this was the view expressed by many respondents about the loss of HIV ringfenced finance. Many of the community-based initiatives were funded from this money and it was generally reported that when ringfencing ceases so would many of the initiatives. Only in one or two cases, where key post-holders (such as a director of public health) had a firm and clear commitment to the area of sexual health, did respondents generally feel confident that the issue would remain fairly high on the policy agenda.

In theory, there are three levels at which alliances can operate. The first involves joint planning and purchasing in which different agencies jointly plan and purchase services from providers according to clearly identified processes of needs' assessments and prioritization. Although the various parties may have different potential resource contributions, they should, in theory, have roughly equal voices in the decision-making process. This model was not found in our fieldwork sites (although some sites were working towards this model). This was probably mainly because of the rapid changes being experienced, but the clearly differing agendas of some agencies do not augur well for the future even when structures have become more stabilized.

The second level is represented by the more commonly found local HIV/AIDS forums, AIDS advisory groups, sexual health steering groups and similar meetings. There were mixed views on these, with the phrase 'talking shops' being used by a number of respondents. Although a range of agencies was represented, many felt that the power to allocate resources remained with a small 'élite' group, and that there was an element of tokenism in the efforts made to hear others' views. The increased feeling of competition inhibited some respondents from contributing as fully as they might. These generally negative views – particularly common among providers – led to strong feelings that these forums were 'yet more meetings' expected of people already under a great deal of time pressure.

The third type of alliance is the less formal level usually known as 'networking'. There were many positive comments received about this level, and many new or planned initiatives were described as arising from the contacts made. Particularly valued were regular meetings of outreach workers, which were described as providing mutual support and encouragement and in making them feel less isolated in their everyday work.

Conclusions

There are a number of exciting and innovative initiatives in the various sites included in this study. However, the conclusion from our analysis of the data was that the planned establishment of strong sexual health alliances was not apparent and we have highlighted some of the reasons for this lack of progress. As recent changes in health and other services have become more established, the situation may be rather less chaotic and uncertain. Recent informal contact with workers in the field, however, suggests that this speculation may be optimistic.

The government's recognition of sexual health as a key target area for the *Health of the Nation* was, in many ways, a welcome (albeit surprising) inclusion. It is, however, ironic that other aspects of government policy on public services may be inhibiting the sorts of collaborative working arrangements which may be necessary if the targets set in the White Paper are to be achieved.

Notes

1   All state-funded secondary schools (for ages eleven and over) in England and Wales are now obliged to publish annual figures showing the proportions of their students who achieved particular grades in public examinations. Newspapers produce 'league tables' of these results and some parents use these as a basis for selecting schools for their children. The increasing competition between schools

for the funding which is 'attached' to students has led to strong suspicions that some schools are basing greater priority on these academic performance indicators than on providing a more 'rounded' education.

2   In 1992, the government published a White Paper entitled *The Health of the Nation*. Five key areas were identified as needing particular attention, including sexual health. Specific targets to be achieved by the year 2000 included halving the rate of conceptions among women aged under sixteen years (from the 1989 rate), and reducing the numbers of new cases of gonorrhoea among men and women aged fifteen to sixty-four years by at least 20 per cent by 1995 (from the 1990 rate). These specific targets were set in the context of more general objectives to reduce the number of unwanted pregnancies and to reduce the incidence of STDs.

3   The study was funded by the Health Education Authority.

4   Since 1987, annual AIDS (Control) Act reports have been required to be submitted by local health authorities. They provide a record of the numbers of new cases of HIV in each area, as well as a breakdown of the probable routes of transmission.

5   Discourse analysis refers to an increasingly popular approach to reading texts. There are a number of 'definitions' used by different authors (see, for example, Potter and Wetherell, 1987; Billig *et al.*, 1988; Hollway, 1989; and Parker, 1992, for discussion of some of the controversies in the area). Our own use of the approach with these data involved paying particular attention to what might be called 'taken for granted assumptions' in our respondents' speech.

6   Recent changes in the National Health Service in England and Wales have encouraged increased needs' assessments in all areas of health. These (in theory) involve detailed considerations of data collated from a wide variety of sources to enable local profiles of need to be produced, so that more efficient evidence-based purchasing can be implemented.

7   Recently introduced changes in the operation of the health service (ostensibly to increase efficiency and effectiveness through encouraging competition) have led to locally based commissions, as well as those in primary care, being given budgets with which to purchase health care. Those actually delivering the service, known as 'providers', need to bid for resources and enter into a contractual arrangement with one or more purchasers. Such contracts contain 'service specifications' which detail the service to be provided and may include, for example, the number of client contacts required per unit of time.

References

ALLEN, I. (1987) *Education in Sex and Personal Relationships*, London: Policy Studies Institute.

BILLIG, M., CONDOR, S., EDWARDS, D., GANE, M., MIDDLETON, D. and RADLEY, A. (1988) *Ideological Dilemmas: a Social Psychology of Everyday Thinking*, London: Sage.

DEPARTMENT OF HEALTH (1993) *The Health of the Nation Key Area Handbook; HIV/AIDS and Sexual Health*, London: Department of Health.

EVANS, D., INGHAM, R. and ROOTS, B. (1994) *Sex Education in Salisbury – Report of an Evaluation in Salisbury Secondary Schools*, Salisbury: Salisbury Health Authority.

HOLLWAY, W. (1989) *Subjectivity and Method in Psychology: Gender, Meaning and Science*, London: Sage.

HUTTON, C. (1992) 'Young people's perceptions', in C. BARON and A. BUTLER (Eds) *HIV/AIDS Sex Education for Young People*, The All-Party Parliamentary Group on AIDS, Occasional Paper No. 3.

NFER (NATIONAL FOUNDATION FOR EDUCATIONAL RESEARCH) (1994) *Parents, Schools and Sex Education: a Compelling Case for Partnership*, London: Health Education Authority.

PARKER, I. (1992) *Discourse Dynamics: Critical Analysis for Social and Individual Psychology*, London: Routledge.

POTTER, J. and WETHERELL, M. (1987) *Discourse and Social Psychology: Beyond Attitudes and Behaviour*, London: Sage.

THOMSON, R. and SCOTT, L. (1992) *An Enquiry into Sex Education – Report of a Survey into LEA Support and Monitoring of School-based Sex Education*, London: Sex Education Forum.

WOODCOCK, A., STENNER, K. and INGHAM, R. (1992) ' "All those contraceptives, videos and that . . .": young people talking about school sex education', *Health Education Research, Theory and Practice*, **7**, 4, pp. 517–31.

Chapter 6

'I Don't Know What I Need to Know': A Peer Sexual Health Project by Young Disabled People

Maura Banim, Alison Guy, Sharon Cahill and Anthony Bainbridge

This chapter reports on a research project conducted in Cleveland, England, which used a social model of disability and peer education to address concerns about young disabled people's access to information and guidance about protective behaviours and sexual health.[1]

The overall aim of the project was to develop an appropriate sexual health promotion initiative for young disabled people. It aimed to utilize a participatory framework wherein young disabled people, working with support from a research team with both non-disabled and disabled members, would themselves devise and deliver this initiative. In order to do this, the project had to reconsider ideas about what constitutes sexual health (aim) and sexual health promotion (process). Diamond (1974) has argued that most concepts of sexual health operationalized in health promotion contain assumptions about 'correct' forms of sexual expression and about norms of performance and expectation. Work in this area has to recognize the diversity in the meaning of sexual health for different people. The sexuality of disabled people is also made problematic and their need for sexual health promotion is seen as being either less or more important than for non-disabled people. Needs differ and diverse education is required that relates to different capabilities, expectations and protective practices.

Integral to the project was the belief that young disabled people themselves must be centrally involved in defining their sexual health needs and developing strategies to meet those needs. Therefore a peer education model was selected as having two key strengths: first, that people are more likely to personalize a health message that may result in behaviour change if they believe that the messenger is similar to them in lifestyle and faces similar concerns and pressures (Sloane and Zimmer, 1993). Second, peer trainers may have their own skills and knowledge reinforced and their self-esteem enhanced through the process of consultation and the exercise of responsibility (Quicke, 1986).

For this particular project, it was critical to be aware that peer education would not necessarily empower the peer trainers. Milburn (1995) argues that peer education can be effective – but to what end? In this area of work, it is easy to transmit, through peer education, the idea that disabled people's sexuality is problematic: that, for example, learning how to avoid pregnancy is as important as learning how to avoid abuse. The agenda and influence of carers and workers can become an unquestioned part of the health message that young disabled people transmit to their peers.

Underlying Values

To ensure the project reflected the agenda and concerns of disabled people, three underlying values were identified. First, Hohmann (1975) has argued that the medical model of disability emphasizes the absence of normal functioning on the part of disabled people and that consequently the issue of disabled people's sexuality is framed within a medical/professional discourse and, generally, within a negative discourse. The project therefore adopted a social model of disability which locates disability in the relationship between people and their social context, and emphasizes the importance of the environmental, attitudinal and social barriers that disabled people face (Oliver, 1984). The social context within which disabled people experience their sexuality thus became a crucial focus, and involved exploring how disabled people can identify and start to dismantle the barriers which prevent them from taking control of their sexuality.

Second, the research began with the premise that young disabled people live in a social context that is complex and contradictory but which must be recognized before effective interventions can be attempted. On one level they face a double jeopardy that can undermine sexual health practices – their sexuality is seen as problematic and they may also have limited access to information and appropriate guidance about sexual health. On another level they also face a double layer of homogeneity. Just as adolescence is often pathologized and homogenized (Warwick and Aggleton, 1990), so is disability. Disability is not necessarily a context which diversifies the experience of adolescence: it can actually be an extra layer of homogeneity – an extra barrier to their individual, diverse needs being recognized. However, while the pathology of adolescence includes risk-taking and activity, the pathology of disability includes tragedy and passivity. This lays open the possibility that the sexual health needs of young disabled people can be perceived by professionals in very different ways depending on the discourse professionals use to frame their client group. Similarly, young disabled people themselves may find difficulty resolving their identity, especially in the context of receiving conflicting messages from those around them.

Third, it has been noted by several researchers and commentators (Morris, 1991; Robbins *et al.*, 1991) that the expression of sexuality within a sexual relationship is one of the 'clearest markers of adult status in our culture' (Heyman and Huckle, 1995, p. 152). Embarking on sexual relationships is generally a precursor to (or at least associated with) more independent living, such as moving away from the parental home. Ultimately the expression of sexuality is linked to the adoption of a number of adult roles that eventually establish autonomy from dependence on one's family of origin. For the most part, this is seen as a natural, if sometimes problematic, process – an essential part of the transition to adulthood which is characterized by the exercise of independence and autonomy.

Obstacles to Transition

There are a number of ways in which the natural transition may be blocked for disabled people. The sexuality of physically disabled people is often pathologized and assumptions are made about their ability, or rather lack of ability, to engage in sexual relationships. The assumption may be rooted in particular perceptions about bodily functioning and the nature of sexual intercourse and/or it may be located in assumptions about attractiveness and desirability (Centre for Educational Research and Innovation (CERI) Report, 1988; Morris, 1989; Shakespeare, Gillespie-Self and Davies, in press). There are also often ambivalent or negative attitudes about the reproductive capacities of disabled people (Morris, 1991; Hasletine, 1993).

The sexuality of people with learning disabilities is also seen as problematic. Heyman and Huckle (1995) argue that most parents or carers see sexual relationships as a 'hazardous' area for the person they support. This hazard is perceived as a lack of ability to act appropriately and responsibly (i.e. in an adult manner) and/or running the risk of exploitation. The belief that the adult with a learning disability could not express their sexuality appropriately leads to a situation where sexuality may not be acknowledged or given recognition. Conversely, the sexuality of learning disabled people may be 'over acknowledged' because it is seen as a natural urge that learning disabled people cannot understand and thus control (Heshusius, 1987).

On a more practical level, physically disabled people (especially younger people with less income, no private transport and limited social networks) may have difficulty getting access to other young people with whom they may form relationships (Anderson and Clarke, 1982). To a large extent this is linked to the 'barriers' model of disability where environmental factors restrict the lifestyle of disabled people (Oliver, 1984). However, it may also be linked to parental or carers' attitudes which include anxiety about widening the social network of the person they support, seeing such social mixing and increased mobility as a potential hazard. Tied in with both these obstacles is the problem of gaining access to information in relation to sexual health. Health services for disabled people are often geared towards the disability and it may be difficult for a younger disabled person to raise an issue like contraception with their GP or specialist (Campion, 1990).

This situation means that it is difficult for many disabled people to achieve autonomy. Ultimately this limits their ability to protect themselves from risks, as it limits their opportunities to gain skills in identifying and meeting their own sexual health needs. In addition to the restricted learning environment, young disabled people may have a poor self-image:

> One of the biggest problems disabled people face is that all the undermining messages become part of our way of thinking about ourselves ... this is the internalisation of *their* values about *our* lives. (Morris, 1991, p. 177)

This exposure to negative constructions of sexuality and the physical constraints facing many disabled people means that young people approaching a sexual health-promotion project may come with ambivalent feelings about sexual relationships or with fears about the consequences of gaining a more positive sexual identity. The delivery of sexual health promotion needs to take account of these issues and cannot be done in isolation from the social context of disabled people's lives.

The Project

In order to achieve its aims, the project set out to recruit and train two Peer Action Groups of young disabled people, one focusing on the sexual health needs of people with physical disabilities and the other on the sexual health needs of people with learning disabilities. The Peer Action Groups consisted of volunteers recruited via interviews from disability projects – day centres, training centres, recreational clubs – in the Cleveland area. Potential recruits heard about the project through letters to various centres, newsletters and personal visits made by the research team.

After recruitment, the participants took part in a training programme to establish a baseline of knowledge in relation to sexuality and sexual health. The training programme also focused on devising a strategy for a sexual health needs assessment which would be carried out by the Peer Action Groups. Following the needs assessment and a presentation of findings to a subsample of respondents (using a rapid appraisal approach based on Annett and Rifkin, 1990), a sexual health promotion initiative was developed.

Recruitment and Training of the Peer Action Group

A total of eight physically disabled people (five males and three females) volunteered to form the Peer Action Group and participated in the training programme. The recruitment of learning disabled volunteers was more problematic. There were a number of concerns from managers of agencies with learning disabled users over their ability to consent. A series of meetings was held to resolve these issues and it was agreed that carer groups should be briefed about the project. However, it was emphasized that consent should be the right of the service user and that centre workers would facilitate this process. Because of the problems in gaining access to learning disabled volunteers, their recruitment was delayed; this chapter will therefore confine itself to reporting on the progress of the physically disabled Peer Action Group.

The physically disabled Peer Action Group received six training sessions, all of which used a participatory approach to establish the baseline of knowledge. The final two sessions explored ways of communicating about sensitive topics and processes involved in data collection to enable an investigation of the sexual health needs of their peers. The evaluation completed at the end of each session and at the end of the programme indicated that the training had been enjoyed and had increased Peer Action Group members' confidence.

Sexual Health-Needs Assessment Initiative

Before the health promotion initiative could be conceived, it was necessary to undertake evaluation research to allow the Peer Action Group to gain an accurate assessment of the issues around sexual health from disabled people from the local area. The Peer Action Group and the research team together devised a strategy for a sexual health needs assessment based on guidelines from Soriano (1995). It was decided to conduct a number of semi-structured interviews with disabled peers and a smaller number of service providers. These interviews would be carried out by members of the Peer Action Group with the research team keeping a record of what was said. After discussion by the group and project team the following issues were identified as being of concern to disabled people and became an integral part of the interview schedule: attitudes to sex and sexuality; sexual health promotion/education already received; areas where further information was required; perceived sexual health needs of self; others' perceptions of sexual health needs; and credible sources to provide information and training. The data generated by the needs assessment and by the rapid appraisal meetings would then enable the Peer Action Group to explore ways of integrating findings into a coherent strategy which would provide the basis for the development of future sexual health promotion initiatives for disabled people.

Findings

The Peer Action Group conducted a total of 72 interviews with disabled respondents over a three-month period. Fifty-six per cent of the sample were male (n = 40) and 44 per cent were female (n = 32) with the age range being between 16 and 67 years. Fifty-seven per cent (n = 41) were aged between 16–35 and 43 per cent (n = 31) between 36–67. The people interviewed had a range of impairments including cerebral palsy, multiple sclerosis, brittle bones, epilepsy and hearing and visual impairment. Some of the respondents had learning disabilities as well as physical disabilities. Fifty-nine per cent of the male respondents lived with parents or carers while only 36 per cent of them lived alone or with a partner. Of the female respondents, 51 per cent lived alone or with a partner and 48 per cent with parents or carers. The remaining respondents lived in residential care.

One of the strongest themes from the interviews centred on the respondents' understanding of representations of sexuality. A number of discourses relating to representations about sex, sexuality and disability arose and most of these were expressed in negative terms. Many respondents were unable to articulate what sex, sexuality or sexual health meant to them. The responses seemed to indicate that some respondents did not understand the questions being asked, while others were unable to conceptualize sex and sexuality. Responses such as 'don't know', 'nothing', or 'it doesn't really mean anything to me' were common. Many people felt they did not know what they needed to know about sex. There was a perception by some that lack of experience was a particularly important element here. They felt that by not having had a close relationship, they were unable to envisage their own sexuality. Lack of knowledge was perceived as an impediment and any knowledge they did have was of little value without the opportunity for exploration. It became clear that many disabled people had adopted a value base which prioritized penetrative sex and this was a crucial aspect of their perception that sex was not for them, as illustrated in the following quotes from two respondents: 'Don't know, it's difficult when you haven't had sex with anyone' (female). 'Don't know about sex, I don't know what I need to know' (male).

A few respondents said their disability had a negative impact on sexuality and sexual expression. Other respondents indicated that disabled people were scared either to ask for information about sex or to have sex. For example, one respondent commented: 'My wife is disabled too so we don't bother' (male). A small group of respondents felt that sex was either not an aspect which was part of their experience (and would not be in the future), or that it was a pathological expression. These responses indicated that sex did not happen to disabled people. 'I think it's a bit disgusting really' (female).

Some of the respondents did have a more positive view of sexuality. A few saw sex as socially desirable and acceptable behaviour. These respondents discussed their sex lives positively and spoke of the importance of being able to have sex when they wanted to. Sex was also seen by some respondents as a positive expression within the context of a close relationship. This sort of response was often linked to traditional ideas about love, trust and closeness as important aspects of relationships, as shown in the following quotes: 'That you were sensible in actions and attitudes towards sex' (female). 'Sex can be about loving relationships' (female). 'Knowing your partner, being aware of partners' wants and what they don't want' (male). Another theme focused on the impact of disability on sexual relationships. It was noted that disabled people's needs and desires were no different from their non-disabled peers but that there could be differences in sexual expression linked to the specific impairments. It was felt that sex was a positive aspect of disabled people's lives and deserved recognition by both disabled and non-disabled people. 'People think disabled people don't do it, but it's only human' (female). 'Safe sex between two people who know each other well enough to get over any hang-ups about disability' (female).

Overall, the needs assessment revealed that for most respondents sex and sexuality were represented and articulated in behavioural terms, there being little mention of attitudes or imagery about sexuality. This could be linked to the lack of positive images or discourses about sex and disability. The messages that seem to be available to disabled people are often linked to a medicalized view of disability that stresses the limitations of impairment (Finklestein and French, 1993) and which may prevent the articulation of a more encompassing sexuality. A further consideration is that, as most of the respondents were living with parents, the development of their sexuality can be impeded or unacknowledged by their carers and by themselves. Lack of opportunity to gain a positive self-image and to attain a sense of their social self seems to mitigate against disabled people's ability to develop positive ideas and attitudes towards their sexuality.

Priorities for Sex Education

The interviews also probed respondents' experiences of sex education in the past and what they thought might be appropriate sex education for disabled people. Many respondents reported that they had received some form of sex education but they qualified their answers, noting in particular the variable quality of this education and the difficulty they had in making requests for information, as this topic proved embarrassing both to them and to those they were expected to ask. Several respondents mentioned that the scope of sex education in special schools was extremely limited. Television programmes and friends were also mentioned and were seen as being credible but inaccurate messengers. Many respondents indicated they did not have anyone with whom they could discuss sexual issues. For example: 'I was very embarrassed when I was younger. I had lots of questions and didn't know who to ask' (female).

Respondents mentioned three main areas of concern. First, many emphasized that both disabled and non-disabled people should have information to enable them to make choices about sexual behaviour. However, it was recognized that many disabled people would require information that was related to their specific impairment. A substantial number of responses were concerned with the need to establish the possible range of behaviours/acts with different levels of functioning. 'We need more specific information, you're just left to get on with that side of life . . . have to learn the hard way' (male).

Second, several respondents felt that having relationships was an important component of sex education but commented that their opportunities to meet other disabled people were limited. This could lead to problems in recognizing the differences between friends and sexual partners and in recognizing the emotional dimension of sex.

Third, many respondents talked about the need for disabled people to be able to protect themselves in sexual relationships. There was a clear recognition of HIV and AIDS and the use of barrier methods to prevent transmission. However, there was little recognition that other sexually transmitted diseases could also be prevented in this way. There were a few misunderstandings over the contraceptive aspect of barrier methods and there was little recognition of the range of contraceptive methods available, although there was a reasonable understanding of their function. Several respondents also mentioned that disabled people needed to be able to protect themselves from unwanted sexual advances.

Most frequently identified as appropriate providers of sex education were 'experts', such as health professionals and teachers. This may reflect a confidence that their specialized knowledge would allow them to offer the specific information disabled people clearly desire. However, it may also reflect a perception that sexuality is a technical/medical issue – which would be consistent with the absence of a more social representation – and/or a recognition that these professionals are gatekeepers to resources such as contraception.

Disabled peers were also mentioned as appropriate deliverers of sex education. It was recognized that they would have valuable insight about the needs and obstacles that disabled people face. There was, however, little comment on their ability to provide specific information. This could be linked to a perception that their peers would face similar problems in gaining information. It could also be a reflection of the way in which disabled people are taught to value non-disabled people, who provide their support, rather than each other (Davies, 1993).

A smaller proportion of respondents identified families as potentially appropriate sources while recognizing the variability of family input on these issues. Some parents discriminated between disabled and non-disabled children in the information they provided and the behaviour they sanctioned. However, a substantial number of respondents strongly questioned the value of contributions from parents and experts. This can be seen as challenging their dependence and the desire of some disabled people to seek information and guidance from an independent source: from people not directly involved in their day-to-day care.

Overall, there was a clear awareness by many disabled people that good quality sex education is vital to promote the sexual health of their peers. It is also apparent that the respondents are not confident about their sexuality and their ability to express it using the knowledge base they currently possess. Those who support these respondents do not currently play an enabling role, although many are viewed as having the potential to do so.

Comparing Perceptions of Sexual Health Needs

The interview also focused on respondents' thoughts about how those who supported them (families, partners, keyworkers) perceived their sexual health needs. Respondents perceived their families as having predominantly negative perceptions of their sexual health needs. This was particularly emphasized by the younger respondents. 'Haven't talked to them, they don't think I have any sexual needs' (male). 'They'd worry how I'd manage' (female). A few respondents noted more positive perceptions which seemed linked either to the strength of the relationship between themselves and their parents or to their own relationship status. 'It's OK 'cos I have a partner' (female). 'My mam's OK but she doesn't know what to tell me' (female). The responses suggest that many parents and carers find it problematic to consider their disabled family member as a sexual being and that, even when they do, they are often uncertain how to offer support in terms of information and in making choices.

When respondents were asked about the responses of keyworkers, the most frequent response was that sexual health needs were not an issue they could discuss. This reluctance to discuss sexual health matters seemed equally shared between the keyworkers and the respondents – and as the relationship progressed it often became more difficult to raise the issue. A few respondents felt that their keyworker would be supportive and helpful if they were ever brave enough to mention the topic.

Another key aspect was the opportunity to access information to help identify and meet sexual health needs. Some respondents had made attempts to gain information but had found this to be difficult: their contacts either did not have the necessary information or questioned whether these were legitimate concerns. One disabled female wanted to know more about *in vitro* fertilization, but past experience made her wary of asking support workers because she felt they would be more concerned with explaining why it was 'unrealistic for her'. Some respondents felt that having a partner would enable them to realize their sexual health needs. This was linked to two factors: that things might become more self-evident in practice or that they would have some solidarity when trying to access information and services.

The perceptions disabled people have in relation to themselves, their families and keyworkers give a vivid illustration of how difficult it is to envisage sexual health needs when there is an absence of a social sexual identity and when sexual identity is defined as deficient in relation to that of non-disabled people. The disabled respondents spoke about having the same needs as non-disabled people, yet in their interactions with these who support them there was little sign that this similarity was acknowledged by carers.

Reflections on the Needs Assessment Exercise

Both the experience of interviewing and the data obtained clearly indicated that disabled people are a very diverse group. There are differences in their knowledge about sex and sexuality, and they have different life experiences and different levels of impairment. Therefore, their concerns about sexual health are different. However, they face a common obstacle because they are regarded as homogenous by many of the non-disabled people who play important gatekeeping roles in their lives (Morris, 1991). Their individual needs and concerns are largely unrecognized beyond the label of disability. As a result, they are presented with similar sets of barriers to the assertion of their individual, diverse sexual identity. The findings reveal that respondents feel they are frequently seen as non-sexual beings, with little acknowledgment of their rights for information about sexual health. The needs' assessment also suggests that disabled people have often taken on board a value base that prioritizes the ability to have penetrative sex and this leaves some feeling inadequate (Diamond, 1974). Specific information about physical impairment and sex is not widely available and, in its absence, disabled people can feel that, because 'normal' sex is difficult, sex is not for them. At the same time, however, the fact that they recognize that there is a need for and right to specific information can be viewed as an assertion of autonomy. However, from a position of being unable to access information it is difficult to identify what you do want and to contest the dominant view.

It is evident that developing and maintaining a positive sexuality is a daunting challenge for many disabled people. If they try to access the positive representations that exist around sexuality they face a set of assumptions that also exclude them. Establishing a positive sexuality also brings the person into confrontation with the misperceptions or denial of powerful others. It is possible to draw parallels with other marginalized groups, such as gay men and lesbians, and to recognize some of the similar restrictions in attempting to meet and mobilize around common oppression (Abberley, 1993). It is not surprising that for many respondents it was more salient to identify negative experiences and hostile environments. In trying to envisage how a positive sexuality can be achieved, disabled people recognize the need to bring these issues into the public domain. There need to be opportunities for disabled people to share their experiences and to recognize that many of the obstacles they face are social in nature and not just a result of their specific impairment. One of the outcomes of the needs' assessment has been a space where respondents can have their experiences validated. Many of the interviews ended with a discussion between the respondent and the disabled interviewer about the shared nature of the experiences noted in the interview.

In relation to sexual health more generally, this research has identified the existence of a dominant discourse of prohibition and risk. Issues of protection (both in terms of safer sex and avoiding abuse) in relation to sexual behaviour were seen as important elements of a sex education programme but were highlighted largely because they were consistent with fearful associations about sex. These representations may be shared by many non-disabled people who find it difficult to regard safer sex as affirmative sexual behaviours (Richardson, 1990; Wilton and Aggleton, 1991). In many people's experience, sex education has served to emphasize sexual practice as dangerous and unhealthy. It may also be that these aspects have been particularly emphasized by those caring for or working with disabled people as further justification for 'not bothering with sex'. If affirmative sexual behaviour is to be promoted for disabled people, much thought needs to be given to challenging the negative representations of sexuality they face. Preparatory work building more positive approaches to sexuality needs to be done with disabled people and those with influence in their lives, before sexual health messages can be usefully delivered and integrated.

The needs assessment interviews imposed a degree of stress on many of those who chose to participate as they covered a potentially embarrassing topic and many interviewees were unused to being asked for their opinions. Interviewers noticed that they often got a good deal of relevant information after the interview schedule had been completed. The findings revealed that there was an implicit agreement not to talk about sex and sexuality. The lack of communication between disabled people and those who support them could be viewed as a marker of independence – a possible assertion of a right to privacy. However, given respondents' frequent wish to access to more information, this is probably not the case. Rather, control of the absence of discourse was seen to be in the hands of carers. Sexual health programmes need to consider the influence of carers' attitudes and how dependency relationships can be renegotiated.

An important dimension of the project has been the process: the construction of a participatory framework which would enable the Peer Action Group to investigate the sexual health needs of their peers and devise appropriate sexual health initiatives. The development of a partnership between the research team and the Peer Action Group was a vital part of realizing these aims. This was a gradual achievement, but at all stages it has been emphasized that, beyond the initial training, the project would involve joint decision-making. Various factors have facilitated the development of partnership: having a clear structure to the project so that the Peer Action Group members could plot their own progress; tangible and intangible recognition of the value of their time (such as contracts, payments for their time, allocation of a budget for the training initiative, mutually convenient meetings, recognizing skills and expertise); and ensuring Peer Action Group members had the lead role in the needs assessment interviews. There were constraining factors to building a partnership and these were largely linked to time constraints and the limited opportunity for the Peer Action Group to meet independently of the project.

Partnership was an evolving process, with the Peer Action Group taking increasing amounts of responsibility. However, their experience of carrying out the needs assessment helped them to recognize that merely offering training or information to disabled people is of limited value if powerful others do not share their perception of disabled people's right to a sexuality.

Conclusions

Most of the disabled people involved in the project, whether as members of the Peer Action Group or as respondents, have a functional knowledge of HIV/AIDS. However, it is difficult to claim that they have personalized this information. It becomes clear that most disabled people do not feel they own their sexuality and do not feel able to take responsibility for it. The Peer Action Group members identified a series of core values which they felt should underpin sexual health promotion. First, disabled people's sexual health must be part of a framework of rights if it is to avoid being ignored or pathologized. Second, the transfer of good quality knowledge into protective behaviour can only be properly accomplished if disabled people are afforded the opportunity to develop interpersonal skills, such as being able to challenge the effects of stereotyping in relation to their self-esteem and body image. Third, gatekeepers who control access to services need to be aware of the particular obstacles and barriers disabled people face and ensure their services are accessible. As part of this, regular consultation with disabled people is essential to ensure that service priorities develop in ways that reflect users' priorities. Finally, the role of families, carers, friends and the wider community is critical. The rights, feelings and effort of all groups should be respected and the focus should be on how to work positively together to develop the sexual health of disabled people. Health promotion interventions around HIV/AIDS, no matter how good the content, will be of limited value unless they recognize and address the immense difficulties disabled people face in trying to claim and take control of their sexual identity.

Note

1   The project was funded by the Northern and Yorkshire Health Authority.

References

ABBERLEY, P. (1993) 'Disabled people and "normality"', in J. SWAIN, V. FINKLESTEIN, S. FRENCH and M. OLIVER (Eds) *Disabling Barriers – Enabling Environments*, London: Sage.

ANDERSON, E.M. and CLARKE, L. (1982) *Disability in Adolescence*, London: Methuen.

ANNETT, H. and RIFKIN, S. (1990) *Improving Urban Health*, Geneva: World Health Organization.

CAMPION, M.J. (1990) *The Baby Challenge. A Handbook on Pregnancy for Women with a Physical Disability*, London: Methuen.

CAMPLING, J. (Ed.) (1981) *Images of Ourselves: Women with Disabilities Talking*, London: Routledge & Kegan Paul.

CANDESIS, M.F. (1991) 'Evaluating the quality of health education programmes', *HYGIE*, **10**, 2, pp. 40–5.

CENTRE FOR EDUCATIONAL RESEARCH AND INNOVATION (1988) *Disabled Youth. The Right to Adult Status*, Paris: Organization for Economic Cooperation and Development.

DAVIES, K. (1993) 'On the movement', in J. SWAIN, V. FINKLESTEIN, S. FRENCH and M. OLIVER (Eds) *Disabling Barriers – Enabling Environments*, London: Sage.

DIAMOND, M. (1974) 'Sexuality and the handicapped', *Rehabilitation Literature*, **35**, pp. 34–50.

FINKLESTEIN, V. and FRENCH, S. (1993) 'Towards a psychology of disability', in J. SWAIN, V. FINKLESTEIN, S. FRENCH and M. OLIVER (Eds) *Disabling Barriers – Enabling Environments*, London: Sage.

HASELTINE, F. (Ed.) (1993) *Reproductive Issues for Persons with Disabilities*, London: Paul H. Brookes.

HESHUSIUS, L. (1987) 'Research and perceptions of sexuality by persons labelled mentally retarded', in A. CRAFT (Ed.) *Mental Handicap and Sexuality: Issues and Perspectives*, Tunbridge Wells: Costello.

HEYMAN, B. and HUCKLE, S. (1995) 'Sexuality as a perceived hazard in the lives of people with learning difficulties', *Disability and Society*, **10**, 2, pp. 139–55.

HOHMANN, G.W. (1975) 'Reaction of the rehabilitation team to patients with sexual problems', *Archives of Physical Medicine and Rehabilitation*, **56**, pp. 8–13.

LONSDALE, S. (1990) *Women and Disability*, London: Macmillan.

MILBURN, K. (1995) 'Peer education with young people about sexual health: a critical review', *Health Education Research*, **10**, 4, pp. 407–20.

MORRIS, J. (Ed.) (1989) *Able Lives: Women's Experience of Paralysis*, London: The Women's Press.

MORRIS, J. (1991) *Pride Against Prejudice: Transforming Attitudes to Disability*, London: The Women's Press.

OLIVER, M. (1984) *The Politics of Disablement: a Socio-Economic Approach*, London: Macmillan.

QUICKE, J. (1986) 'Pupil culture, peer tutoring and special educational needs', *Disability, Handicap and Society*, **1**, 2, pp. 147–64.

RICHARDSON, D. (1990) 'AIDS education and women: sexual and reproductive issues', in P. AGGLETON, P. DAVIES and G. HART (Eds) *AIDS: Individual, Cultural and Policy Dimensions*, Basingstoke: Falmer Press.

ROBBINS, B., OWEN, J., MORGAN, J. and STUART, O. (1991) 'From eternal child to adulthood: issues in sexuality and disability', in *The Disabling Society*, Milton Keynes: Open University.

SHAKESPEARE, T., GILLESPIE-SELF, K. and DAVIES, D. (in press) *The Sexual Politics of Disability*, London: Cassell.

SLOANE, B. and ZIMMER C. (1993) 'The power of peer education', *Journal of American College of Health*, **41**, pp. 241–5.

SORIANO, F.I. (1995) *Conducting Needs' Assessments: A Multidisciplinary Approach*, London: Sage.

WARWICK, I. and AGGLETON, P. (1990) 'Adolescents, young people and AIDS research', in P. AGGLETON, P. DAVIES and G. HART (Eds) *AIDS: Individual, Cultural and Policy Dimensions*, Basingstoke: Falmer Press.

WILTON, T. and AGGLETON, P. (1991) 'Condoms, coercion and control: heterosexuality and the limits to HIV/AIDS education', in P. AGGLETON, G. HART and P. DAVIES (Eds) *AIDS: Responses, Interventions and Care*, London: Falmer Press.

Chapter 7

Doubly Deviant? Women Drug Injectors and their Use of Drug Problem Services

Kate Philip, Luan Bruce and Janet Shucksmith

Despite evidence both for high rates of problem drug use among women and for the greater damage done to women by drug misuse, men outnumber women in the use of the problem drug services in Scotland by 2.8 : 1 (Scottish Drugs Forum, 1994). Moreover, accounts of drug use and policy responses frequently discuss the 'drug user' with no reference to gender (Robertson, 1988; Strang and Stimson, 1990; Evans, Sandberg and Watson, 1992). The drug user referred to is, often by implication, male. Alternatively it is assumed that the experience of women is no different to that of males. Thus the specific patterns of women's drug use and the problems inherent in supplying services for this category of need remain neglected.

At a policy level in Scotland, attention has been drawn to the situation in publications such as the Scottish Office Task Force Report (1994) and the Scottish Drugs Forum policy statement on women and drug misuse (1994). Within the Task Force report it is recommended that drug-problem agencies 'review their service for women drug misusers (including childcare needs) (*ibid.*, p. 3). The report goes on to urge services to 'consult their women clients for their views on the services offered and encourage them to be involved in the long term monitoring and evaluation of service provision with the aim of developing a more attractive service to women drug misusers' (*ibid.*, p. 3). However, given the low numbers of women currently using services this exhortation may be unrealistic, at least in the short term.

Women's Lives and Drug Misuse

There is considerable evidence to show that the numbers of women misusing legal drugs is greater than that of men (Nelson-Zlupko, Kauffman and

Morrison Dore, 1995) and that the number misusing illicit drugs is higher than recorded by official statistics (Scottish Drugs Forum, 1994). Moreover, research evidence would seem to show that the onset of drug misuse in women is more frequently associated with trauma (Kane-Cavaiola and Rullo-Cooney, 1991), that substance-abusing women experience higher levels of guilt, shame, depression and anxiety about their addiction than men (Reed, 1985), and that women experience more detrimental physical consequences of drug use at lower levels and in a shorter amount of time than men (Doshan and Bursch, 1982).

Overall, women drug users are viewed as socially deviant in not conforming to dominant images of appropriate behaviour for women (Barnard, 1993). Kohn (1992) has suggested in a history of drug-taking in Britain, that hysteria about drug-taking in the wake of the First World War was strongly linked to fears about the changing role of women and expressed in terms of how drug-taking was one example of how respectable if misguided women could be drawn into depravity through becoming independent. Contemporary accounts of women drug takers would seem to perpetuate this enduring theme.

Henderson (1991, p. 266) has pointed out how judgements about women as 'nice' and 'bad' have mediated care responses to women drug injectors. In turn, this 'triple layer' of stigma leads to women losing self-respect:

> These dimensions of social stigma were reflected in the experience of women infected (with HIV) through drug use in that they expressed a greater sense of shame (particularly where prostitution had played a part in funding drug use) taking the blame upon themselves.

Women who inject drugs are usually regarded as 'vectors of infection' in relation to HIV. This is even more likely to be the case if they have been involved in prostitution, as early accounts of HIV infection suggest. The importance of maintaining a *decent* (i.e. non-promiscuous) image has been a means of regulating women's behaviour in the wider social context, and drug-taking women who are labelled as promiscuous face particular condemnation (Ettore, 1989). Women who are pregnant or who have parental responsibilities may be particularly discriminated against in their day-to-day dealings with others in the community and with professionals – and defined as feckless. Literature on women drug users has focused almost exclusively on their reproductive role, as Taylor (1993) indicates in a recent review.

Thus the needs of women in their own right command little attention and their needs are often unquestioningly assumed to be similar to that of male users. This perspective can be linked to patterns of discrimination against women in the wider community and has been challenged by feminist analyses such as that by Ettore (1989) and more recently Taylor (1993). Taylor (1993) has pointed out the relative paucity of sociological research into how drug use fits into the lives of women in a recent ethnographic study of injecting drug users in Glasgow. One exception to this overall tendency is a study by

Barnard (1993) in Glasgow which highlights the reluctance of drug-injecting women to make use of needle exchanges.

This chapter explores some of the dilemmas facing women drug users who may require specific kinds of service in relation to their drug use through an account of a study undertaken in 1994 in Aberdeen. Three hypotheses are outlined and explored. The importance of appropriate forms of research and investigation are discussed. We conclude with a discussion of the implications of the findings for policy and practice.

The Study

This chapter reports findings from a collaborative study carried out in the Grampian Region of Scotland by the Department of Education at the University of Aberdeen and Drugs Action Aberdeen, a voluntary organization which, among other services to drug users, provides a needle exchange in the city centre. This study, funded by the Grampian Health Board, was in part a replication of a study carried out by Hart *et al.* (1991) in London. Although Grampian Region is currently characterized by low reported HIV-prevalence rates, these have risen steadily in recent years. In January 1995 there were 89 known cases of HIV infection in the Grampian Region as compared to 1052 in the Lothian Region which includes Edinburgh.

The study comprised two phases: first a survey of HIV-prevalence and behaviours among injecting drug users in Aberdeen who were clients of the Drugs Action needle exchange. Sixty of the 124 clients who used the needle exchange at that time participated in the study, of whom fifteen were women. Thirty-one clients were not invited to take part since they were new referrals, so the response rate represented 75 per cent of those eligible to take part. All volunteers gave a saliva sample and participated in an in-depth interview. None withdrew from the study. In the second phase of the study interviews were conducted with a more hidden population of injecting drug users who were not currently in contact with the Drugs Action needle exchange.

In phase one the low level of participation by women was notable. This, combined with the findings that women were more likely to use the agency when they were injecting heavily and, like younger injectors, were more likely to admit to engaging in risky sexual practices than older or male injectors, had prompted a concern to focus on women in the second phase. To this end, every effort was made to recruit women to the second phase of the study. Time was spent with outreach workers in different neighbourhoods and with sex workers in the red light area of the city. A wide range of contacts was established and followed up with community-based organizations, women's groups and youth projects. Although some of these contact points were unsuccessful in recruiting women, they provided valuable data highlighting the stigma faced by women who admit to injecting drug use. Some staff were unwilling to acknowledge that clients were injectors, since this would breach confidentiality; but for others the main reason was that the organization in question had a strict anti-drugs policy which would mean withdrawing services to clients known to be injectors. In some cases this policy meant staff would 'turn a blind eye' to signs that someone in their care was an injector, while others conceded that some injectors are highly skilled in concealing their drug use (Bruce *et al.*, 1994).

In the second phase, despite these extensive efforts to reach women who did not make use of the drug agency, the ratio of male to female users in the sample remained substantially the same. Sixteen women participated out of a sample of 83. Nevertheless, the second phase in-depth interviews elicited some telling data on women's feelings about the services available to them and their reasons for not using existing drug services. In addition to questions about their patterns of drug use and sexual behaviours, respondents were asked to comment on their responses to existing service provision.

The Working Hypotheses

Three possibilities emerge as potential explanations for women's lack of visibility in this context. These are not mutually exclusive but it will be useful to explore them as starting points in order to highlight some of the particular needs of women and the implications for service provision.

One potential explanation for women's invisibility is that they are adept at concealing their drug use because they manage their habit effectively and succeed in adapting their drug use to the rest of their lives. They are able in the main to remain stable and in control of their habit. They deploy considerable skill in avoiding services and managing their drug use within their lives. Women may not even acknowledge or recognize that they are problem drug users. Being able to conceal their drug use and control it to the extent of being able to 'keep the place' as regards family, community and work, minimizes the need for services. Thus this population may remain comfortably hidden.

An alternative explanation might be that women are isolated by their own fears about disclosure and consequent loss of reputation if their drug use was to become known. Such fears force them into dependency on male partners to provide supplies, information and services, and they only approach services when this conduit breaks down in some way. Lack of self-esteem and lack of autonomy may further inhibit women from seeking out services and this powerlessness may be manipulated by male partners. Moreover, reliance on partners may symbolize important aspects of the relationship.

Linked to the above, but a distinct hypothesis, is that agencies themselves are unable to meet the everyday needs of drug-using women who are then forced into depending on specialized services only when triggered to do so by crisis. Agencies have enough difficulty in fulfilling the needs of existing users and the women they tend to see are partners of existing users who often appear to require similar forms of service. Drug agencies may also tend to view female partners simply as partners rather than as users themselves. This view may be compounded when women adopt a self-managing role, presenting themselves as less 'out of their faces' than their partners. Thus services which, on the face of it, exist to provide support may unwittingly marginalize and stigmatize women drug users.

Keeping it to Themselves – Women as Managers

I've managed to keep it to myself. My folk don't know so I wouldn't risk going in there.

Clearly, there are fewer women using drugs agencies than men. Findings from phase one of this study (Bruce *et al.*, 1994) show that in contrast to male users of Drugs Action, women appear to use the service when they are already injecting heavily, and many female occasional users appear to get their injecting equipment elsewhere. A very small number of the women who participated in phase one of the study presented a confident and 'hard' front, simply coming in to use the needle-exchange service and leaving, having little contact with the staff or other users. The remainder of the sample were women who were clearly there on the basis of their relationship with a male partner. This led the research team to focus more intensive efforts on contacting women for the second phase of the study.

In the second phase, initial contacts were made with a wide range of agencies and community groups, drug-problem services, GP surgeries, pharmacists, community workers and day centres where staff agreed to cooperate and to invite women to participate. In addition to the issues raised in reaching women, further questions were raised about how truly voluntary such involvement might be: for example, if there was a suspicion that participation might be linked to favourable decisions about a prescription, women may have felt a subtle pressure to take part.

Findings from phase two further reinforce the evidence that stigma and fear of the social consequences of being identified as a woman who injects drugs was a major concern in how services are perceived. Many women went to considerable lengths to protect their anonymity as these quotations suggest: 'Going into DA would be too visible. Women get too embarrassed about people knowing they inject.' 'Needle exchange in a chemist is too visible and women especially get embarrassed about injecting.'

For many women, the need to keep their drug use private was reinforced by wider societal expectations about appropriate female behaviour. Many held traditional views about their role and had internalized critical views about their own deviance which in turn reinforced feelings of low self-worth and esteem. Their often considerable success in retaining their independence was rarely recognized by themselves and the impression was given that this was a precarious anonymity, subject to change at any time.

The need to keep their practices secret also affected how women viewed professionals, as with this young woman in talking about pharmacists: 'Some of them are pains in the arse and ask loads of questions. It depends who serves you. The pharmacist himself is usually nice.' The following woman wanted to have minimal contact with an agency, viewing attempts to involve her in any way as a potential threat, and she remained alert to any attempts to engage her in conversation. 'I'd rather go to a chemist. They (DA) would ask too many questions – too chatty. I don't want to talk about my drug use to strangers.'

For women who were responsible for children, this reluctance was even more apparent and resulted in some ambivalence. Concern for their children might be a factor in deciding to seek help, but alongside this ran an awareness of the risks of triggering unwanted interference or even losing their children into care if they looked for help from agencies. Social workers were viewed with particular suspicion by mothers who feared that knowledge of drug use would be perceived as evidence of neglectful mothering, thus reinforcing a finding by Green and her colleagues in Glasgow that social work departments were identified as agencies which confiscate children (Green *et al.*, 1993, p. 330). There may be a number of reasons for this: social workers are perceived as among the most powerful professionals with whom women were likely to come in direct contact but clearly they have not been successful in allaying the fears of this population. Whatever the reason, there seemed to be less overt suspicion of health and housing visitors, although they were also mentioned less frequently.

Such fears operated at a local level, too, as anxiety was expressed that neighbours or even ex-partners might take disapproval further by 'grassing' to the authorities. Several men also identified this as a reason for women not disclosing their drug use. For some men the resultant reliance on them by their female partners may reinforce their power in the relationship by allocating them a role as provider. This often provides a substitute identity to that of breadwinner or worker, for example. By contrast, there was little concern about how their role as a father would be perceived by professionals, as the following quotations from interviews with men show. 'Women with kids would be scared it gets back to their social worker and they would be seen as unfit mothers.' 'Women might be scared their kids get taken away if folk know they inject drugs.'

· Thus there was evidence that women do reject services for fear of damaging their reputation since such involvement is perceived as posing a threat to their anonymity and is thus potentially disruptive of their lives. Far from being a positive choice, then, for some women this determination to remain hidden appears to derive from the perception that the risks of such involvement outweigh the benefits. These women tried to use services on their own terms by adopting strategies which resulted in minimal contact and which enabled them to maintain a low profile. Their use of services was thus purely instrumental as they rejected attempts to provide additional information and advice. Nevertheless, it is important to acknowledge that many women succeeded in managing their habits effectively: they continued to live and work in the community and retained their anonymity. One participant, for example, had been unaware of the existence of the agency but would not have approached it anyway: 'I didn't know about it when I was using a lot 'cos I kept my habit hidden. Now my drug use is under control . . . and I'm doing OK.'

Like a number of women in the study, this participant saw herself as measured in her drug use in contrast to some of the men whom they observed to be self-indulgent and chaotic, taking little responsibility for themselves or their actions. Those women who were most public about their drug use were seen to be those who had no children and those whose responsibility for their children was temporarily suspended as their children were already in local authority care. In some ways this group had perhaps little further to lose as their drug use had been defined as problematic by the authorities and action had already been taken.

Hunting and Gathering: Men as Gatekeepers

A lot o' women have kids and get their needles from their lads because they don't want their kids taken into care.

For some women, this fear of public visibility resulted in a reliance on male partners in a number of ways, not least to find and provide supplies. Most women in the sample had been introduced to injecting by a male partner and this had a powerful impact on the relationship. This in turn reinforced already low levels of self-esteem and self-agency among some women. Male partners were endowed with a high level of trust and sometimes optimistic hopes that they would be discreet about a partner's drug use. A number of men made efforts to reinforce the dependency and this took a variety of forms. For some men this 'provider' role was an important element of the relationship, according them a sense of identity in 'taking care' of their partner and family. For others it offered a means of developing a traditional male role for themselves and boosted their self-esteem. The opposite was true for those women who felt they could not afford to alienate male partners and were trapped by being unable to access services on their own behalf.

Evidence of the filtering of information by these male gatekeepers was also present: restricting information about the existence of women's sessions provides an example. This gave males considerable power over their partners because they acted as filters of information and as negotiators on their behalf with individual agencies. Clearly for many women this power imbalance compromises their ability to challenge partners if they are dependent on them for supplies: 'I get my boyfriend to get works for me.' 'There's a few (pharmacists) I use. Others look at you funny. He gets them usually.'

With few exceptions, male participants in the study, even those who had girlfriends who injected, described women drug injectors as 'mingin' (a local term meaning 'dirty') or 'slags'. Such contradictory attitudes were puzzling: it is clear there were some differences between public statements and private relationships with some men protecting the reputation of their partner by vociferous denials that they were injecting. The assumption that women are 'vectors of disease' underlay many of the statements made by men. This paradox has been noted in a number of studies in relation to HIV infection: people distance themselves by making exceptions in relation to those they know and trust (Ingham, Woodcock and Stenner, 1992; McKeganey and Barnard, 1992).

Nevertheless, the role of 'gatekeeper' was clearly a familiar one to men in the study, bringing with it some form of identity as the provider for a partner: for some this became a version of the 'hunter and gatherer' theme. For example, one woman in our study was the main breadwinner through working as a prostitute, but she remained under the control of her partner who attempted to control her drug use by securing supplies, organizing her drug-taking activities and offering her 'protection' on the street. This involved him 'keeping an eye *on* her' i.e. hanging around when she worked as a prostitute, which she interpreted as pressure to earn money to support both habits. He in turn described this as 'keeping an eye out *for* her' – ensuring her safety while she was working – but he was nevertheless anxious to secure her money as quickly as possible. The distinctions between these interpretations of this situation are important ones in highlighting how women are disenfranchised by such dependence on male partners.

The 'gatekeeper' role was clearly demonstrated in one incident where the researcher had arranged to interview a young woman after she had collected her prescription at a pharmacy. When she emerged from the shop, a man approached her and tried to lead her away. She apologized to the researcher and moved away with him. A further example of the pressure such a role can exert on women was provided when a couple arrived at the agency when it was only open for a women's session. The young woman elected to join the session much to the annoyance of her male partner who hung around outside for the duration of the session, knocking on the door from time to time and asking her to leave with him. His main fear was that the group were discussing him.

Meeting Need – Agency Roles

I didn't want people to know I was on drugs. DA is very public.

Clearly many drug agencies, despite good intentions, are hampered in their efforts to provide services to women. Many are perceived by women as not just offering inappropriate help but as making it difficult to protect their reputation as 'decent women'. The locations are too public and being seen there would be risky in itself. For some women, other users of agencies were viewed as posing some risk to them or their children. 'I know a heap of bams (idiots) who go in there so I don't like to go in. They're not people I'd like to be seen with.'

For some, using services was viewed as incompatible with other areas of their lives and the desire to keep away from 'undesirables'. Stereotyped images of other drug users were also commonly cited: 'I have a child and am at college so I don't associate with those people.' 'This is a safe one [referring to a particular pharmacy] – but it costs money to get here. The one nearer had people outside trying to buy your script off ye.'

Lack of childcare at facilities was a recurring issue for women. But for some this was linked to other clients' attitudes and behaviour. 'There's naebody to look after the bairns. DA's not a place for bairns. You don't want to take your bairns into contact with other drug users.' But for women with children there was also a need expressed to have some time to explore their concerns as women rather than mothers. This is an issue women articulated with some diffidence, which perhaps illustrates how easily the needs of women drug users are conflated with that of their children. 'If you've got kids you don't want to trail them with you. You need a crèche with toys. Kids can stop you from having a conversation if they're crying.' 'You can't talk to someone when you've got a bairn screaming.'

Moreover, many drugs agencies are seen as projecting a macho image which may in itself inhibit women from seeking help. This may be a process which is both subtle and complex, drawing staff into colluding against involving women in the agency in a variety of ways: men may be more directly demanding of attention by challenging workers' decisions and policies, or by dominating space and worker time, as well as by 'slagging off' women. The need to retain and work with those young men who are perceived as high risk and who behave this way may be at odds with providing a safe environment for women. Thus sexist behaviour and remarks may go unchallenged, or those workers who do resist such stereotyping may feel unsupported or ridiculed. Reluctance to be seen as open to accusations of being 'politically correct' may also inhibit the development of interventions to address women's needs. Beliefs that this arena is 'unsuitable for women and children' may serve to reinforce feelings of uneasiness and 'not belonging'.

Outreach work focused solely on the 'street' and in public spaces may unintentionally further marginalize those women whose social networks revolve around localized neighbourhoods. At a more subtle level, workers may themselves consider women to be 'doubly deviant' and therefore resistant to making services more 'user friendly' for women.

Many women in the study specifically identified their needs for some service provision but were unsure how these could be met. Sex workers expressed the need for a drop-in and related services. Other specific requirements were also identified as remaining unmet by existing provision: 'A rehab would be good especially for women who've got kids and can't go off to Liverpool or London.' It is clear, however, that many women could not envisage an agency or service which would or could meet their needs. Was this because the existing models were so far from meeting their requirements that they found it impossible to imagine how slight adaptations or extensions could come to help them?

Conclusions

In describing data from this study, three possible reasons were suggested for women's current low levels of use of existing drug agencies and services. These three explanations overlap considerably, but it is clear that the specific needs of women themselves – rather than simply women as carers of children – need to be better understood before effective services can be designed.

Clear parallels exist between the difficulties in accessing women for research on such topics and in devising appropriate strategies for service provision. It may be helpful to explore some of these in relation to the findings outlined above.

> What we do know is that although need does not necessarily equate with hard to reach, many of the easier to reach individuals contacted by prevention services are probably less in need of such services than those who remain hidden to even the most skilled and adept of outreach workers. (Rhodes, 1994, p. 93)

Similar difficulties in accessing women injecting drug users are apparent in research terms. In addition to the difficulties posed above, there is some need to examine the inadequacy of existing research methods. Classic forms of survey research are often limited to sampling frames of identified users and may thus do little more than describe the absence of women using service provision. Qualitative techniques have often relied on 'snowballing' sampling techniques to reach hidden populations. But for women who are making it their business to remain hidden not just from the authorities but also from the community, this technique is deficient. Modifying it in the manner adopted by Taylor (1993) who accessed individuals and relied on them to introduce and 'vouch' for her to others, is highly demanding in terms of the skills of the researcher in building up trust and empathy with whole networks, and may only be feasible within an ethnographic framework.

Accessing women through their male partners may be problematic or even counter-productive: some men, as we have noted, may have a vested interest in retaining control over their partners. Using such an approach may serve to reinforce women's dependence on their partners and their low self-image. In this study, a number of male respondents offered to encourage their partners to participate. However, no women were recruited through this approach. In addition, some women who were partners of known inject-ing drug users were recruited through other channels. Similarly, there was evidence that male injecting drug users, despite their offers, were not passing on information to partners about women's sessions at the agency. Male part-ners may have a vested interest in retaining control over their partners and some examples of this have been cited. In another instance, a young man who was vocal in condemning women drug users as slags and boasting that his partner would never be seen 'at the harbour' was met at the harbour by the researcher. He maintained he was just waiting for a friend but he accepted a number of condoms and it was clear from the statements made by other sex workers working in the area that his partner was working as a prostitute, and he was waiting for her to return from being with a client.

Those women who do make use of services may have to adopt strat-egies that mark them out as 'exceptional' in terms of ignoring attempts to marginalize them from the service. It is clear that for many women fears of becoming visible arise from efforts to protect their reputations in the wider community. Thus Scottish Office exhortations to women to become involved in the monitoring and evaluation of services may demand considerable pre-paratory work in preparing the ground for women to make use of services on their own terms.

A model suggested by Rhodes (1994) for outreach work looks promising on the face of it, since it moves from a focus on the individual to a recog-nition that drug users, like others, do not operate in a social vacuum and that there is a need to address contextual factors. Clearly for many drug users finding money, housing and childcare may be of a higher priority than reduc-ing the risks of HIV infection. Rhodes emphasizes the need to take account of these in the design of outreach work, stressing the importance of finding ways of empowering drug-using networks at a collective level. However, there are serious difficulties in seeing how this can be adapted for groups of women. How is community created in the first place? How can it be sustained in the light of many women's fears about becoming visible? For women in sex work there are clear precedents for recognizing community norms as Taylor and others have suggested, but this may be an infinitely more difficult prospect in isolated housing estates. In a recent study of women who are HIV-positive in East London, Feldman (1995) found that women wanted services to be sited not in their own borough but in a neighbouring one where they would be less visible and less open to discrimination or attack.

The planning of services to women drug injectors therefore has to take into account the complexity and subtleties of the patterns of discrimination against women in the wider society and to explore how these are reproduced and interpreted within drug-using cultures. This entails a rigorous rethinking of methodologies of assessing need and demand and a reconceptualization of how to access and work with hidden populations.

References

BARNARD, M. (1993) 'Needle sharing in context: patterns of sharing among men and women injectors and HIV risks', *Addiction,* **88**, pp. 805–12.

BRUCE, L., SHUCKSMITH, J. and PHILIP, K. (1995) *HIV Prevalence and HIV Awareness of Injectors Not in Touch with Drugs Action's Needle Exchange,* Report to Drugs Action and Grampian Health Board, Aberdeen: Department of Education, University of Aberdeen.

BRUCE, L., SHUCKSMITH, J., PHILIP, K. and PILLEY, C. (1994) *HIV Prevalence and Awareness of Users of a Needle Exchange,* Final Report to Grampian Health Board, Aberdeen: Department of Education, University of Aberdeen.

DOSHAN, T. and BURSCH, C. (1982) 'Women and substance abuse: critical issues in treatment design', *Journal of Drug Education,* **12**, pp. 229–39.

ETTORE, B. (1989) 'Women, substance abuse and self help', in S. MACGREGOR (Ed.) *Drugs and British Society,* London: Routledge.

EVANS, B., SANDBERG, S. and WATSON, S. (Eds) (1992) *Working Where the Risks Are: Issues in HIV Prevention,* London: Health Education Authority.

FELDMAN, R. (1995) Paper (n.t.) presented at the Social Aspects of AIDS Conference, October, London.

GREEN, S.T., GOLDBERG, D.J., CHRISTIE, P.R., FRISHER, M., THOMSON, A., CARR, S.V. and TAYLOR, A. (1993) 'Female streetworker-prostitutes in Glasgow: a descriptive study of their lifestyle', *AIDS Care,* **5**, 3, pp. 321–35.

HART, G.J., WOODWARD, N., JOHNSON, A.M., TIGHE, J., PARRY, J.V. and ADLER, M.W. (1991) 'Prevalence of HIV, Hepatitis B and associated risk behaviours in clients of a needle exchange in central London', *AIDS,* **5**, 5, pp. 543–7.

HENDERSON, S. (1991) 'Care: what's in it for her?', in P. AGGLETON, G. HART and P. DAVIES (Eds) *AIDS: Responses, Interventions and Care,* London: Falmer Press.

INGHAM, R., WOODCOCK, A. and STENNER, K. (1992) 'The limitations of rational decision-making models as applied to young people's sexual behaviour', in P. AGGLETON, P. DAVIES and G. HART (Eds) *AIDS: Rights, Risks and Reason,* London: Falmer Press.

KANE-CAVAIOLA, C. and RULLO-COONEY, D. (1991) 'Addicted women: their families' effect on treatment outcome', *Journal of Chemical Dependency and Treatment*, **4**, 1, pp. 111–19.

KOHN, M. (1992) *Dope Girls: The Birth of the British Drug Underground*, London: Lawrence & Wishart.

MCKEGANEY N. and BARNARD, M. (1992) *AIDS, Drugs and Sexual Risk*, Buckingham, Open University Press.

NELSON-ZLUPKO, L. KAUFFMAN, E. and MORRISON DORE, M. (1995) 'Gender differences in drug addiction and treatment: implication for social work intervention with substance abusing women', *Social Work*, **40**, 1, pp. 45–54.

PERRY, L. (1979) *Women and Drug Use: An Unfeminine Dependency*, London: Institute for the Study of Drug Dependence.

REED, B.G. (1985) 'Drug misuse and dependency in women: the meaning and implications of being considered a special population or minority group', *International Journal of the Addictions*, **20**, pp. 13–62.

RHODES, T. (1994) 'HIV outreach, peer education and community change: developments and dilemmas', *Health Education Journal*, **53**, pp. 92–9.

ROBERTSON, R. (1988) *Heroin, AIDS and Society*, London: Hodder & Stoughton.

SCOTTISH DRUGS FORUM (1994) *Policy Statement: Women and Drug Use*, Glasgow: Scottish Drugs Forum.

SCOTTISH OFFICE HOME AND HEALTH DEPARTMENT (1994) *Drugs in Scotland: Meeting the Challenge*, Report of Ministerial Drugs Task Force, Edinburgh: HMSO.

STRANG, J. and STIMSON, G. (1990) (Eds) *AIDS and Drug Misuse*, London: Routledge.

TAYLOR, A. (1993) *Women Drug Users: An Ethnography of a Female Injecting Community*, Oxford: Clarendon Press.

Chapter 8

Sexual Début and the Risk of HIV Infection among Young Gay Men in Norway

Anne-Lise Middelthon

Whether young gay men are at heightened risk of acquiring HIV infection is assessed differently in different countries and studies. Several studies in the USA, for example, highlight young gay men's particular risk for HIV (Ekstrand and Coates, 1990; Hays, Kegeles and Coates, 1990; Kelly *et al.*, 1990; Lemb *et al.*, 1994). Project SIGMA in Britain, on the other hand, found no difference between young and older gay men's participation in sexual practices which involve the risk of HIV infection (Davies *et al.*, 1992). In Norway, knowledge on this subject is limited. Epidemiological surveillance, however, gives no indication of young gay men being at higher risk. By the end of 1995, only two men under the age of 20 who had had sex with another man, had been found to be HIV-positive. Among those 45 men diagnosed as having HIV infection in 1995, one man was in the age group 20–25 years and four men were in the age group 25–29 years. The rest were aged over 30 (Nilsen, 1996).

The issue of young gay men and risk has been discussed in Norway by the Gay Men's Health Committee and The National AIDS Team on a number of occasions in recent years. The research project, from which findings are presented here, was initiated as a result of these discussions and is based on the following premises. First, independent of whether or not studies from the US and England and Wales have shown unambiguous results, efforts to transfer their findings to the Norwegian situation are problematic. Second, more and better knowledge on the subject is needed. Finally, regardless of whether young gay men are more or less at risk than older men, issues associated with being young and gay demand specific attention.

The study was carried out in three Norwegian towns: Oslo, Trondheim and Bodø in collaboration with the Norwegian Gay Men's Health Committee. A qualitative methodology was adopted. Over a period of 22 months, twenty self-identified gay men, aged 17–22 (mean age 19.5) were followed through repeated (3–5) in-depth interviews lasting 2–3 hours. A general interview guide was developed for the initial interview, while subsequent interviews were planned individually. The first interviews were conducted during March 1994. Data from the interviews were complemented by focus-group discussions with adult gay men and young men other than those being interviewed. So far, two focus groups have been conducted in which 22 young men have participated.[1]

The project's link to an ongoing epidemic makes it imperative for the dissemination of knowledge gained to be an integral part of the research process. As soon as judged appropriate, therefore, analyses and results are conveyed both to the Gay Men's Health Committee and its local branches, and to the National AIDS Team. Because dissemination is followed by discussion in which reactions, opinions and experiences are put forward, the dissemination process itself becomes part of the data-gathering and verification process.

When entering the study, the participants had already had their first sexual experience with another man. This makes it possible at this stage in the research process, to examine the nature of this début and related topics of possible relevance for HIV-prevention. The focus in this chapter is on the sexual début itself. Allied processes of 'coming out' or 'self-acceptance' as such are not a theme for this study. Experiences from, as well as the categorization of, the sexual début will be explored, as will the issue of how or whether sexual début is 'scripted', the possible consequences of a relative absence of script for the sexual début, and the strategies adopted to compensate for such an absence. In order to investigate and analyse sexual début, Simon and Gagnon's analytical concept of 'sexual script' will be used. The focus here is on the cultural and interpersonal aspects of sexual scripting. Scripting at individual level will not be discussed. Thus 'sexual script', as the concept is used here, does not refer to intrapsychic scripts but to scripts existing between or among people.

The Sexual Début and Sexual Scripting

In Gagnon and Simon's (1973) early work on sexual scripts, two major dimensions of scripts are described. The first deals with 'the external, the interpersonal – the script as the organization of mutually shared conventions that allows two or more actors to participate in a complex act involving mutual dependence. The second deals with the internal, the intrapsychic, the motivational elements that produce arousal or at least a commitment to the activity.' (*ibid.*, p. 20). Subsequently the collective dimension of 'cultural scenarios' has been introduced. These provide instructions on the cultural level about how persons should and should not behave culturally (Simon and Gagnon, 1986). The cultural scenarios in which we live provide the basis for and shape our sexual behaviour and encounters, while interpersonal scripts offer concrete information about and facilitate the sexual encounter. They also delineate what is permitted and expected in a given sexual encounter. The intrapsychic script, on the other hand, 'facilitates the emergence and persistence of individual motivation to act in a sexually significant way' (Simon and Gagnon, 1987, p. 366). Cultural scenarios, interpersonal and intrapsychic scripts provide three analytical levels, but are dynamically interactive in the practice of social, cultural and mental life (Gagnon, 1990, p. 10). Different scripts influence one another and often presuppose each other. For example, the script for gender roles is of significance for, and learned prior to, the development and acquisition of sexual scripts. Simon and Gagnon (1986, pp. 98–104) emphasize that all human behaviour is in some way scripted and that scripts 'are essentially a metaphor for conceptualising the production of behaviour within social life'. They emphasize that the very concept of the scripting of sexual behaviour implies a rejection of the idea that the sexual represents a very special or unique quality of motivation.

Sometimes directly and openly, but just as often indirectly and hidden, the cultural scenario instructs us how to feel and act. The cultural scenario is the basic source for the creation of scripts and 'provides qualities of instruction that make most of us far more committed and rehearsed at the time of our initial sexual encounter than most of us realise' (Simon and Gagnon, 1987, p. 365). When living in a 'heterosexual culture', however, this will not be the case for a homosexual man.

Abelson (1981) has drawn attention to what he calls 'meta-scripts'. These are generalized as opposed to specific scripts and do not prescribe concrete behaviour in specific situations in the way that specific (e.g. sexual) scripts do. The script for the relation between an experienced and an inexperienced person may be seen as one example of a meta-script and will be applied here in the discussion of the relationship between the experienced and the inexperienced in the context of sexual début.

Sexual scripts are not static. A glimpse into changes in scripting may perhaps be gained from an examination of attitudes towards women and condom use. When the HIV epidemic began, the sexual encounter in which a young woman initiated condom use was only vaguely, or not at all, scripted; the traditional gender-role script, saying that girls are not to act as sexual subjects, took precedence. This led young women who demanded or suggested condom use to be categorized as 'loose' or 'whores' (Middelthon, 1992). In Norway we can now see the contours of a process evolving towards the development of an interpersonal script in which the initiation of condom use by women is both scripted and given a positive value.

Laws and Schwartz (1977) have analysed scripts in relation to female sexuality and also discuss the prevalence of sexual situations which are not scripted, weakly scripted or only scripted in subcultures or segments of societies. As an example they use the lack of a script for a woman propositioning another woman. No woman learns a script like this during her early socialization. If she does not belong to a group where such scripts are available, everything will be left to her individual innovation. For young men beginning a gay life, the situation may be similar. In contrast to heterosexual young people, knowledge about sexual début and what it involves is not generally available to young gay men, since it is not culturally scripted. A script provides knowledge about what will or what is supposed to happen during the début. This makes the situation predictable to some degree, and provides the neophyte with a possibility of having at least some feeling of control. Among the young men who took part in this study, the lack of such a feeling of control is striking, as is the absence of script for the début.

Categorizing and Scripting the Sexual Début

Before discussing how participants experienced their sexual début, some differences in the way homo- and heterosexual young people categorize sexual début will be explored. The way the sexual début is categorized forms part of the début, and a closer look at it may contribute to a better understanding of this kind of sexual encounter.

Début refers to something being done for the first time. Sexual début refers to an act associated with sexuality being done for the first time. In doing something for the first time, a change in status occurs – the transition from being a person who has never done a particular act to becoming a person who has. Along with the acquisition of status as a person who has 'done it' follows the knowledge of what 'it' is.

Before a transition which is characterized as début, the neophyte will possess no knowledge about the life event in question which is based on their own experience. If knowledge is to be gained in advance, it must be acquired through secondary sources, given that such sources exist and are available. For heterosexual young people, secondary sources about sexual début exist. Despite the fact that quality and relevance of the sources may vary, factual books, as well as fiction, lyrics, films and pictures, are easily available. Talks about what will, or what is supposed to, happen during the début, together with stories about how it was, form part of the ongoing discourse about sex among heterosexual young people. This discourse is not dependent on whether or not the sexual encounters discussed are part of the young people's experience, or even on whether they have happened at all.

For the homosexual début, secondary sources are significantly fewer and often experienced as non-existent. Knowledge or information on homosexual début is not generally available through easily accessible sources like books and films. Neither is the homosexual début part of the dominant discourse on sexuality among young people. Before their first sexual experience with another man, few young gay men will belong to or participate in a gay community or friendship group. If they had had such an attachment it might have provided access to information and possibilities for taking part in, or listening to, talks or discussion about the homosexual début.

In Norway, the heterosexual début is marked by the first experience of vaginal penetrative intercourse and accordingly does not refer to a person's first sexual act or encounter, but to a specific sexual act that is culturally defined as début. The definition of heterosexual intercourse is taken for granted to such a degree that a more specific term than début or 'first time' will seldom be needed. What 'début' refers to is common knowledge which is understood immediately. An illustration of this is found in Norwegian scientific articles on heterosexual début (Kraft, 1990; Pedersen, Clausen and Lavik, 1990). Here the term 'sexual début' appears in the title of these articles without further specification. Only on careful reading does it become clear that the sexual début referred to is in fact vaginal intercourse. From the choice of title it seems that, consciously or unconsciously, the authors assume that the term début is sufficient to make the potential reader realize what the article is about. The authors are probably right in their assumption that there is no need to state that the content is exclusively about heterosexual vaginal penetrative intercourse. This will automatically be read into the title.

Participants' Characterization of their own Sexual Début

Data on their first sexual encounter and début was gathered from all the study participants. Often a story about the sexual début or first sexual encounter was shared independent of, or before, specific questions on this subject. Those participants who did not bring it up themselves were all asked what experience or event they regard as their début. The answer came promptly except from two participants. One specific experience was already categorized as début. However, what sort of experience or event was described as début varied strongly. Mads, one of the two young men who found it difficult to answer, said he started to have sex with another boy when they were 14 years old and continued for two years and so 'eventually it must have become a début'. While Yngve was not capable of singling out one particular event 'because everything flows together'.

Arild, by way of contrast, did not hesitate for a moment when asked. He counts the first time he had sex with another man as his début; the activity was mutual masturbation. Hans offers a different appraisal of what qualifies as début:

> The first time I was with a boy was when I was between 3 and 7 years old. We played doctor and that kind of thing. I have always known that I was gay. The boys I was together with from 12 to 14 were jerking off friends, and sucking also, but not kissing. Sucking was more towards the end of it, and with one particular boy. If you kissed then you were boyfriends. When I was 14, I found out that I had to stop

all that, and started having a girlfriend. We had sexual intercourse and used condoms Then I got a boyfriend.

To be sure I had understood him correctly I asked again what he regards as his début. Hans answered: 'When I got a boyfriend and we both knew. That we were gay I mean. I was 16 . . .' thereby imbuing a sense of authenticity to the event he defines as début. Steinar expresses himself this way:

> Not with the boy I played with as a child. Not before third grade in secondary school and then it was with a girl, we had sexual inter-course. I lay with a man before that, but then I felt exploited. I was 19 years old.

Steinar distinguishes the latter event from others by placing it in a category other than sexual début, namely exploitation. For him the absence of ex-ploitation becomes one criterion differentiating his categorization of début. 'When I first had an orgasm, I was 12. Afterwards I taught the others.' This is Frederick's definition of début. For David, his début involved lying close to a man and hugging and being hugged. Lars, on the other hand, did not see himself as having had his début before having had anal intercourse. Months before he had had a relationship with another gay man, 'but we only kissed and masturbated. It is the first intercourse, that's my début. I have never thought of what happened earlier that summer when I have been thinking about my début.'

Gerhard also answers immediately and says he can identify one specific event as his début, but he does not remember exactly what happened:

> I have thought a lot about it. I don't know. I have forgotten every-thing I did at that time. But I know that it was the year I was 15. Everything happened that year. I was good at repressing things. At that time, they just disappeared afterwards. I forgot everything. I had to forget otherwise I could not function. But I know it was all inno-cent, not oral sex or fucking.

A range of sexual events are therefore categorized as début: the first sexual encounter with another man regardless of the sexual act performed; the first sexual encounter with another man who also identified himself as gay; the first act of penetrative intercourse regardless of the partner's sex; the first act of anal intercourse with a man; the first time of lying close to another man who was also gay; the absence of exploitation; or the first time of having an orgasm. In their categorizations, the participants excluded or did not men-tion playing sex games with other children, when they themselves were chil-dren, and masturbation together with other boys during puberty. Even if no shared idea of what qualifies as sexual début can be seen, one feature clearly emerges: namely, the existence of a distinct event categorized as début by the participants themselves. What kind of event qualifies for this classification depends on subjective assessment. Only the outer framework of the category is pre-given. The event judged significant by the person in question constitutes the content. It is, however possible that when some young gay men link their début to penetrative intercourse, this linkage expresses an adaptation to the dominant script for the heterosexual début rather than subjectively felt value. That all but two participants categorize one particular sexual event as their début may be seen as an expression of the internalization of, and adaptation to, a cultural convention saying that in sexual life a transition called début exists.

It may be argued that as a category, heterosexual début is restricted and closed whereas homosexual début is unrestricted and open. Open here refers to the availability of space permitting the subject to let what is important to him form the basis of his categorization. On the other hand, this 'openness' may be more an 'emptiness' reflecting the lack of scripts for homosexual début as well as a lack of recognition of homosexuality. May be in the future, a category will be scripted which provides real space for the individual to let what is important to him signify the transition. Or perhaps the category of sexual début will lose its meaning and evaporate.

Experiencing Sexual Début

The sexual début as discussed here involves another person. Generally he is either of the same age and with about the same sexual experience, or he is older and significantly more experienced. Four of the twenty participants fall into the category of those who had their sexual début with someone their own age. The material is too limited to draw general conclusions about the situation in Norway. In England and Wales, Project SIGMA found that 39.4 per cent of gay men involved in the study had their first homosexual experience 'with someone who was within a year of their own age; rising to 48.1 per cent for within two years' (Davies *et al.*, 1992, p. 264). But first homosexual experience does not necessarily refer to the event held as début.

The experiences of those who had had their début with someone their own age will be discussed before those who did so with an older and more experienced partner. Emphasis in the subsequent discussion is on the latter group.

Début with Someone of Same Age

Among those who had their début with someone their own age, two kinds of relationships were found. The first appears among those whose first sexual

experience had been with another young man who did not identify himself
as gay and perhaps expressed contempt for gay men like Mads did:

> I had a sexual friend from when I was 14. It was masturbation, suck-
> ing and intercourse. It went on till I was 15, I saw it as experiment-
> ing, he was not gay. I had a guilty conscience because I felt nothing
> for him. It was only to satisfy myself that I was with him. He even
> started to talk about girls while we were doing it. I did not wanted
> to kiss, neither did he. Kissing is the most personal thing.

Mads felt trapped, as his sexual desire could only be met in a relationship
which he could not at the time justify to himself. Not having positive feelings
for the other man was experienced as painful, as was the idea that sex should
become an aim in itself.

Among those who had had their début with a man of the same age we
also find relationships that were described as good and close. Claus had such
a relationship.

> I met him in secondary school. We had been to a party. We went into
> a cottage, locked the door and lay down under three feather quilts
> and all those things. Then he said 'it is so nice to be scratched on
> the stomach'. Extremely exciting, also what happened beneath the
> belly. Not very much did happen, but it was all very strong.

On the whole, precautions against HIV were not taken at the time by members of this group. They felt that HIV had nothing to do with them. Despite
the fact that these sexual encounters hardly involved any risk of HIV infection, the level of fear that imbued young men's descriptions of their lack of
precautions is striking. Some encounters were described as if they were in
themselves infectious, independent of any virus. Safer sex did not become an
issue for this group before they started to have sex with a man other than
their first partner.

Début with a More Experienced Partner

Among those making their sexual début with a partner more experienced
than themselves, the partner also tended to be older, but except for two partners, less than 35 years of age. Many of the participants and those who took
part in focus groups expressed the feeling that even if the début was nothing
special, 'to have done it' was in itself very important. In one of the focus group
discussions, strong doubts were even raised about whether it was possible to
find anybody 'who felt that the first time had been all right'. When describing
his début, for example, Arild expressed himself like this:

> I was 19 and had no images of what was going to happen. I was picked
> up, I would never had dared to pick up someone myself. I went home
> with a man, what happened was kissing and mutual masturbation.
> When we had finished he pushed me out of the door. It was not a
> good experience. But I could say to myself, 'now I have done it'.

Arild's experience of not having any idea or notion of what was going to
happen was common. As his sexual début, Frederick described his first orgasm. Here, however, I will describe his story about the first time he was with
a man for the purpose of having sex. They had met via a hotline and Frederick
had agreed to meet him. After meeting in a bar, they went back to the
man's house.

> I ended up spending the night. When we were about to go to bed,
> he became like an animal. I didn't manage to say no, I felt that I had
> to take part in anal intercourse, that it was a part of it. I knew
> nothing and thought that if this is how it is, this is how it is. It really
> got me down.

Condoms were not used and Frederick says he did not think of it at all. They
met several times the following week. The same thing happened again, and
again Frederick says he did not manage to say no to anal intercourse, 'because I thought this was how it was supposed to be. But it was painful and
I did not want it. It was not only he who was active, I liked it better when
I was the active one.' Condoms were not used during this week either and
Frederick comments:

> I did not think of HIV during the whole week. I don't think HIV was
> in my head as something that had anything to do with me. HIV and
> AIDS were more like atomic war, hunger and other things which are
> in the world but have nothing to do with me.

Why he thought that anal intercourse was a necessary part of the encounter,
he explains like this: 'He was in a way above me, it had to do with age and he
had more experience.' Frederick describes his situation as a snare in which
the unequal distribution of power is determined by knowledge, experience
and age.

Ivar, too, says he did not think of HIV at the time of his first sexual
experience and that he had no images of what was going to happen:

> It was someone I met before he who became my boyfriend. I met
> them both on a hotline. He was in his twenties and came in a car.
> When I met people on the line and agreed to meet them I always
> told them to come to a place where I could see them before making
> contact. This had happened several times before this time. I went

home with this man. What we did was sucking, jerking off and kissing. I did not think of HIV, but when I read about it afterwards I became very frightened. I was 15 and afraid all the time I was with him. I had no idea of what was going to happen the first time, I had not read much pornography either, only in straight magazines that friends had.

Eivind also described the other man as the one possessing experience and knowledge, but he experienced this as a good thing. He said he is good at setting limits, but not a talker. Since his words are few, he gives signals with his body. During his début, his experience was one in which his partner showed responsibility. Eivind claims this

is how it is. It must be so, because it cannot be otherwise . . . the one who is older and experienced takes the initiatives and the younger one signals when he doesn't want to continue.

For him this functioned well and he reported feeling good to 'be allowed to be the younger one'. Experiencing sexual pleasure, however, was felt as threatening. When we first talked about his début he describes it like this:

I was picked up by a man who asked if I would go home with him. I did not really understand what I agreed to. It gave me very little. I signalled that I did not want intercourse or sucking. That was easy.

When we returned to describe his début later in the interview he goes back on his earlier claim that he got little out of it and says:

I had an odd feeling afterwards. Something wasn't right. I kept thinking that this was not what I wanted. I denied it having been good and imagined it as awful, rather disgusting. The feeling that it had been good didn't last long and it took more than half a year before I again could stand the thought that it had been good.

Hans, too, had a début where he was pleased that his partner took the lead:

We had sex the first time we met, but he liked only safe sex. I had met a vanilla type. It was only nice, sucking and massage, no penetration. When I look back at it now I understand that he gave me a gift by letting me start in that manner, and I know now that he did it very very consciously. But at that time what occupied me was that he should be in love with me and how terrible it was that he was not.

Lars argues that older or more experienced partners tend to take advantage of young men's desire to feel loved:

I had started to call the hotline. In the beginning I only listened and it was a real relief when I started to talk. When I was 19, I talked with a man, got his number and called him back. We talked several times before I went to see him. I think I was taken advantage of then. I was very keen. When you are 19, setting limits is not easy. It was not clear to me what was going to happen. I was to sleep in his guest room, but then he said that if you are nice and pretty you may sleep in my room. That was taking advantage of me, I fell deadly in love with him. It was the only time we were together, he excused himself afterwards. We had unsafe sex, anal intercourse, I was the passive one and he did not use a condom. I was very innocent. I felt that when he said that I might sleep in his room if I was nice and pretty, then I was ugly if I was not allowed. I had not been thinking of anal sex at all. I think I just let it happen. I was very passive. I did not suck and I think there was very little kissing too.

Because many respondents described their first experience of anal intercourse as physically painful, and several never managed to go through it, I asked Lars whether it had been painful:

It is very strange, but it was not painful. The strangest thing was that I was not afraid afterwards. I trusted him. I thought that he does not have HIV. I pushed it away. I think that an adult has more responsibility. In the beginning the young are tempted. They are picked up by older experienced men who know what to say to flatter them sky high. I had never been given compliments before. It is different for straight people. With us it is more quick and crazy. The one I was with, I think he knew he had a responsibility he did not take.

Christopher believed, as did Hans and Lars, that his partner had been in love with him and felt it hard when he discovered that this was not the case. But in relation to HIV, he felt in control and had felt no fear of infection:

I used a condom when I sucked him. We talked about it and I said I wanted to take no chances. He sucked me without a condom because he liked it best that way. We tried anal sex too. I had dreamed about it, but I was too tight. I always use a condom. I had heard about HIV long before I knew I was gay and have always carried condoms with me.

Jan had his sexual début when he was 20 years old. He had planned it carefully and felt safe as Christopher did:

'I was in Oslo where several places tempted me. I was tired of waiting, it had to be done. At Enka [a gay club] I picked out one that looked

nice and kind and went with him to his hotel. He was 40. It felt good
that he was that old, others would have been more like myself; too
clumsy. We had anal sex, sucked and jerked off and we used condoms.

When asked whether they had talked about using condoms, Jan answers:

I said when we left Enka that 'Oh! I must take some condoms.'
Someone had told me that there was a bowl of condoms at Enka.
Then he said 'So you want me to use a condom.' We did not use
condoms on so-called dry sucking. Maybe that was a bit foolish, but
I thought no more about it. I did not want to see him again. He had
not understood that it was the first time for me. So I said he should
not have a guilty conscience about that and that I had gone out to
pick up a man.

I asked Jan what he had thought it would be like:

It was in the back of my head that this was how it was supposed to
be, with fucking and things, I had images of that. Afterwards I have
found out that fucking is not such a big need for me. I know now
that I do not want to have anal sex before I am in a stable relationship. It is after all a very intimate thing.

In the focus group discussions, it was generally agreed that the experienced
partner is usually the oldest of the two, but also that it is experience rather
than age that determines who is most in power. Power resides in the one who
knows most. 'The début is a learning situation and in such a situation it is
the experienced who decides.' It was forcefully claimed that if the experienced one does not want to use a condom or have safer sex, little can be
done by the inexperienced one. 'I thought that he is older than me and
surely knows how it is to be. You don't ask for condoms then. You think that
he knows best. I didn't really have a say in that matter.'
      In one focus group where everybody commented on this, only one young
man said that he would have used a condom the first time regardless of what
the other person wanted.

On Using Meta- or Generalized Scripts

Young gay men are in limbo when it comes to the availability of sexual scripts.
The ecclesiastic meaning of the concept limbo signifying the place where those
stay who, through no fault of their own, are denied access to heaven, probably
best describes the situation. The question arises, what kind of alternatives are

to be found in this liminal state? One strategy to compensate for the lack of situationally specific scripts may be to utilize non-specific or meta-scripts, another the translation of a heterosexual script into a homosexual script or, as was often seen, a combination of the two.

The meta-script for the relation young/adult or inexperienced/experienced could be seen in the situation of almost all the young men who had their début with an experienced partner. This script is in many ways a teacher/ pupil or apprenticeship script, ascribing responsibility and leadership to the more experienced partner.

When the question of power relations was brought up in the focus groups it was strongly argued that it is the experienced partner who is in power and decides. Power arises from experience and, during the début, it is taken for granted that along with power and experience comes responsibility. It was also felt that the only option for the inexperienced partner is to trust the one with more experience and knowledge. Eivind felt it cannot be otherwise. He claimed that during the début, the experienced partner will always be the one who takes the initiative, while the young man is supposed to signal stop when, or if, he does not want to go any further. Hans and Eivind also felt it good to be in the position of an apprentice and to leave leadership and responsibility to the partner. When the situation was not felt good by some of the others, it tended to be because the partner did not live up to the young man's expectations.

It appears that in the younger partner's eyes at least, the experienced partner does not often realize that the younger places him in a teacher's position. Some of the début situations involved unsafe sex. It is possible that what for the young man seems an abrogation of responsibility is viewed differently by the experienced partner. He may have made a sober calculation of the risks involved. Based on knowledge about his own HIV status and the low probability of the younger man being infected, he may have judged using a condom or practising safer sex to be an unnecessary precaution. Such reasoning does, however, lack reflection on his role in the sexual encounter, and does not take into account the possibility that he may be met with special expectations. For the young men who later discovered that their partner had judged them to be HIV-negative, this was frightening. Since the young men associate condom use with responsibility, lack of condom use became an expression of irresponsibility. This was so, even if showing responsibility is exactly what the experienced partner felt he did.

The association between condom use and responsibility and safety was generally shared by the young men interviewed (Middelthon, 1996). To encounter negative attitudes towards and/or lack of condom use during early sexual experience may be unfortunate. How the partner behaves in the sexual encounter is of significance for the young man's acquisition and development of knowledge and scripts, but the consequences may go beyond this. For the young man, the experienced partner represents being gay, an identity he is about to acquire. In this situation the experienced partner, in a sense, becomes the generalized gay man. If he is seen in this way and distorts the young man's notion of responsible behaviour and how you treat other people properly, it may hamper his process of self-acceptance. This, in turn, may influence his possibilities for protecting himself and others – a phenomenon Lars phrases like this: 'It is difficult to have safe sex if you have no self-respect.'

For some who left responsibility for safer sex to the experienced partner, it may not solely represent lack of knowledge or scripts but also a contempt for, or complicated attitudes towards, their own sexuality. Feeling contempt for one's own sexuality may make it difficult to act on desires and wishes, or to be proactive in the sexual encounter. By leaving the lead to the other, there is a distancing from the sexual act and the act becomes something the partner does to you. Contempt, or lack of respect, for one's own sexual feelings and acts can also make it difficult to set limits.

> If it is not nice what you do, then it becomes difficult. Then it is so, that if you have said A, you have to say B. When it's not nice what you do, then it's very difficult to make yourself precious. (Gerhard)

When adopting an apprentice script for the sexual début, mechanical modelling constitutes one way of implementing the script and learning the practice:

> Before I started I had no idea about how gay men had sex. In the beginning there were those who told me and those who didn't. They did something – I did the same. It came automatically. He does this – I do after. The idea that I could think of something myself did not strike me at all. At least not in the beginning and when it comes to HIV you have to trust the one you are with. (Per)

It seems as if the experienced partner at times may overestimate the young man's knowledge of HIV. The young men have good general knowledge about HIV, but may feel insecure when the knowledge is to be transformed into practice. This is specifically so for oral sex. Because authority is ascribed to him, the experienced partner needs to consider carefully the possibility of the young man drawing possibly erroneous conclusions about the risks of HIV transmission from the way he acts.

Heterosexuality as Baseline

Many of the participants claimed they had no clear notion of what was going to happen during their début. Even though the sexual desire and longing for love was strong, corresponding images did not develop from this. Perhaps just because the emotions are strong and at least partly experienced as forbidden, they are suppressed before surfacing as conscious pictures. Even if they have no clear notion about what is going to happen, some knowledge is possessed by the young men. The scripts for heterosexuality and its début are known, and form a baseline for the development of sexual expectations with other men, however vague they may be.

Before beginning this project I knew that homosexuality does not necessarily involve penetrative intercourse. But I did not acquire this knowledge before I started to do HIV-related work in 1985. At that time, a colleague, to his surprise, noticed that many of us, his colleagues, linked homosexuality closely to anal intercourse. It was necessary for him to enlighten us. Not before being confronted with his rejection of this image did I realize I held such a notion. Through subsequent discussions, I learned that this is an idea shared by many. Though not explicitly formulated, implicit is the idea of the homosexual encounter as a version of the heterosexual encounter. The young men interviewed displayed a similar thought operation, when they used the heterosexual encounter as a baseline for sexuality as such.

In the traditional script for the heterosexual encounter, the grammar is clear. The man is supposed to be the subject as the woman is supposed to be the object. Roles and sequences are fixed in a predetermined pattern in which penetrative intercourse is the ultimate goal. If applied directly to the homosexual encounter, the syntax of the heterosexual script will prescribe that the final act should be anal intercourse. Davies and Weatherburn (1990) discuss this subject and argue that safer sex is more difficult to negotiate and less likely to occur in an encounter where the sequences are fixed and the power distribution unequal. They argue that the subject/object relationship, typified in the traditional heterosexual script, is counter-productive for negotiating safer sex.

It may be argued that if a person fully surrenders to the already fixed grammar of a script or schema, he deletes himself as a subject. Jan did not delete himself as a subject during his début, but he did not escape the grammar of the heterosexual encounter. Jan planned his début carefully and during it he initiated and practised safer sex. Nevertheless, he was overruled by the grammar of the heterosexual encounter as he held images of anal intercourse as a prescribed and fixed part of the sexual encounter. Later, he learned that it is not necessarily so and made his decision to postpone having intercourse, as for him 'fucking is not such a big need'.

Something analogous are the experiences described by another participant. After having said he had had heterosex as a model Richard explains: 'It is easy to think jerking off, sucking and then fucking. It is easy to just switch from the hetero films.' This is a direct translation of the heterosexual script and its grammar – a grammar which Stian had learned from gay porn magazines: 'I got an idea through porn magazines, first you should suck and then comes anal fucking, then you did the right thing. I thought that everybody had anal sex.'

Several of the participants made the comment that the Norwegian Gay Men's Health Committee in its work focuses too much on anal sex:

> They are too occupied with anal fucking. Everybody thinks that everybody does it. It was too much. I felt that one ought to have it. I guess it is so because they are concerned about HIV. But they say when and not if you should have anal intercourse.

Frederick, too, brought up the issue that many think fucking is necessarily part of sex:

> I had such a period myself when I had anal sex without really wanting it. That is why I have been eager to find out if others have experienced it the same way. After having talked with a number of other young gays I think many have. First a sudden start with anal sex, and only then cosiness and thereafter finding one's own level.

Frederick's observation fits well with the data of this study. Many take the traditional heterosexual script for granted and time is needed to learn that sex does not necessarily include penetrative intercourse. In a process like the one Frederick describes: the first counter-reaction may be a total rejection of anal sex. The choice, then, is still determined by the heterosexual script, as the strategy adopted here is a direct negation or reversed version of this script. A next phase is hopefully one in which the individual develops and acquires a script which does not carry with it a fixed or cemented grammar, but allows the subjects to decide on the basis of what is right and good for them, as long as this is also true for, and does not harm, their partners. For many this will include anal sex as one option in the repertoire. In their discussion of perspectives on fucking, Davies *et al.* (1993, p. 127) draw 'attention to the fact that anal intercourse plays an important part in the sexual repertoire of many gay men'.

> It would seem that unsafe sex occurs when desire is articulated through a rehearsal of domination rather than a celebration of equality. (Davies and Weatherburn, 1990, p. 122)

To fully be a subject in one's sexual life demands a lot. Among other factors it demands a suspension of the traditional script for heterosexuality. Since the emphasis here is on the problematic issues linked to the sexual début situation, the period following the début seems to be different. There are certainly exceptions to this, but what seems to emerge is a picture of young gay men in the process of developing scripts that allow for and prescribe equal or subject–subject relationships within which safer sex is the norm and also generally practised. Built into being a sexual subject certainly lies the possibility of choosing to be an object. These are issues which will be subject to further investigations.

On Separating Sex and Love

In Norway, sexual behaviour is supposed to be an expression of love, and not to be enjoyed just for the sake of pleasure or as an expression of friendship (Kvalem and Træen, 1995, p. 83). This attitude is certainly not necessarily matched by practice, but it constitutes part of the general scripting of sexuality in Norway. It is striking how wounded many of the participants felt when they found that their partner did not necessarily link love and sex. Most were unprepared for the possibility of separating sex and love, and felt it painful to find that sex could be seen as an aim in itself. The term 'cynical' is repeatedly used to describe the feeling. Many fall in love with the man they have sex with the first time and feel betrayed afterwards when they discover that the partner 'had not meant anything more'. The longing for love and intimacy is often just as strong as the sexual urge, and separation of the two is felt by many initially to be impossible.[2] To interpret and understand the partner's reactions and behaviour is difficult. Nice words are easily taken as expressions of love, as are sexual interaction and initiatives.

Some time later, the feelings are still strong about this, but participants nevertheless emphasized that they do not think their partner deliberately deprived them of the knowledge that love was not involved. Instead, many argue, as Christopher does, that regardless of whether or not he now better understands why it was the way it was, 'he [the partner] could likewise have looked back ten years to remember what it had been like'. A paradox may lie hidden here. It is possible that the reason why the experienced partner does not place himself in the position of the inexperienced is because the situation is all too familiar. If so, empathy may be felt to be threatening, because pain and agony are embedded.

On the Bracketing of HIV

'It is easy to push HIV into the background when there is so much else you have to manage.' During the period surrounding sexual début, factors other than lack of scripts may contribute to such a bracketing of HIV. Pre-AIDS studies of the process of coming out shows how this process can be painful and severe, but also carries with it the potential for positive changes in the life of the individual (Plummer, 1975; Coleman, 1982). More recently, coming out in the area of AIDS have been discussed by Rotheram-Borus, Hunter and Rosario (1994, p. 163) who point out that 'Coming out appears to be a difficult and stressful process for lesbian and gay adolescents growing up in a homophobic society'. How painful or severe this process becomes depends on a combination of political, social, cultural and individual factors.

Coming out has not been an easy process for the participants in this study:

only two of them experienced coming to understand that they were gay as 'natural and without any problems'. The rest have all gone through difficult, and even tormenting, processes of self-acceptance, and some denied being gay at times. All those involved in the study have come to terms with being gay. Despite this, while many express feelings of joy at being who they are, just as many still struggle with anxieties and worries. However, all expressed the view that coming out was easier than they had expected and that great improvements had taken place in society. Nevertheless, they also experienced that prejudices against, and contempt for, homosexuality still exist. Only one of the participants says that in school, he received good education on sexuality which also included good education about homosexuality.

Plummer (1975, p. 133) sees 'lack of clarity of signs' as one of the characteristics of the 'status passage to homosexuality as a way of life'. This lack of clarity of signs is still a problem, not only in the début, but also in the period surrounding it. The sexual début is often concomitant with the time when the young men start going to places where gay men meet. This new world is hard to interpret if one is unfamiliar with the codes. This in itself causes stress and tension. In addition to the problems of the coming-out process, come HIV specific issues and questions. If they have not already done so, the young men will, during this period, come to understand that they will find their partner(s) in parts of the Norwegian population where HIV, statistically, is more prevalent than it is in most other segments of society. And they will learn that HIV is something which, in one way or another, will influence part of their sexual life from now on. HIV is closely linked to semen. In contrast to heterosexual men, gay men will not only deliver, but also receive, semen. Half of the participants held ambivalent attitudes towards semen which was felt to be poisonous and disgusting. The message that semen is potentially deadly inside the body but safe on the body surface can thus be difficult to understand and hard to believe in. Long-term emotional work may be needed to come to terms with this.

There are therefore many factors making sexual début a difficult life experience and which result in some men bracketing HIV in order to get through it. Young men who do not feel comfortable with the way the sexual encounter develops may nevertheless feel that their only option is to trust their partner, throw themselves into it and take whatever might come. Not in situations of physical force, they could have chosen to leave, but choose to stay. 'To do it' or 'to have done it' is urgent and imperative.

Stian explained how he feels that exposing yourself to danger at one point in time may be protective in the long run:

> I believe many do it like this, they just let things happen. You yourself are only a tiny part of it, it is the one you are with who is of importance. You may meet a person who knows that he has exposed himself to HIV but who tells you to relax and that there is no danger. If it is like this, you risk being helped to gain confidence in yourself which is very important, and at the same time being in danger.

Next time we met he continued on this issue: 'It is sometimes necessary to take some chances and maybe expose yourself to danger in order to be able to protect yourself later.' Seen from a health perspective, such a strategy might be considered irrational, while understood in the right context it makes sense and reveals an immanent logic. Annick Prieur (1988) describes situations in which making choices which involve unsafe sex make good sense subjectively.

Conclusions

'Being young' is not, and cannot be, treated as one uniform, fixed or unchanging period in life. Many processes, stages and events varying by time and context, as well as in significance and impact, constitute this period. In this chapter I have focused on one event only: the sexual début. During the sexual début or very first phase of sexual life, young gay men may be vulnerable to exposure to HIV. In the début situation, the inexperienced expects the experienced to take the lead and show responsibility. If the experienced partner does not initiate or does not wish to use condoms, asking for this can be very difficult. Before the début, clear notions or images of what is going to happen are held by few. As no 'sexual script' exists for the characterization of the homosexual début, no 'script' exists for its performance. One strategy to compensate for this absence is to act according to the script for the heterosexual encounter; another to validate the script for the relationship between inexperienced and experienced. The strategies are often combined. Regardless of whether the début is experienced as good or not, 'having done it' carries an urgent value of its own, which may result in a bracketing of HIV-related concerns.

Even if significant transformations have taken place in Norwegian society, a lot has still to change before gay men can start their sexual life under acceptable circumstances. Despite formal acceptance and recognition from society, young gay men are still met with prejudice, contempt and discrimination. The way the educational system deals with the issue of homosexuality is one example of this. Homosexuality is still not an integrated and central part of education on sexuality. This lack of genuine recognition in society is also mirrored by the absence of generally available scripts for young men who start their sexual life. Since its first plan of action against the HIV epidemic, the Norwegian Board of Health has repeatedly emphasized the need for changes in the educational system as well as the importance of such changes for the prevention of HIV (Helsedirektoratet, 1986, 1988, 1990). Neither this, nor 1981 legislation which made illegal discrimination based on sexual 'disposition, way of living or orientation', has led to the changes needed.

But changes are not only needed at the societal level. While the Gay Men's Health Committee will contact few young men before they start their sexual life, the experienced partner is reached by their work. The sexual début is not an act involving one person alone. Nevertheless, when sexual début is discussed, it is often as if the experienced partner disappears. Perhaps this is so because the event is unique to only one of the two. But if the début is to be safer for young gay men, the experienced partner needs to come forth more clearly as an active presence in this encounter. If he does so, he may contribute to the young man's development of a feeling of control, free from fear or danger.

Not all young men feel confident in their knowledge of HIV. HIV-related material therefore still needs to be visible and available in places where gay men meet. Frederick, who did not think of HIV during the first week he had sex with a man, was later made to realize that HIV had something to do with him by an HIV poster at a gay club. When developing materials, we should take into account the fact that young men will also be an audience, whether or not they are the target group.

The Gay Men's Health Committee in Norway is currently giving priority to efforts aimed at increasing the experienced partner's awareness of the role he plays and the expectations he is met with. Increased emphasis is being given to work to reach the young men as early as possible. But if we are to avoid, or substantially limit, the occurrence of début situations that involve the risk of HIV transmission, of increased fear or self-contempt, it is crucial that efforts are also taken at the societal level.

Acknowledgments

The young men participating in this research shared their experiences, emotions and reflections with great seriousness and generosity. Without their contribution, this study would certainly have been impossible. The Gay Men's Health Committee is a good and inspiring collaborating partner. The National AIDS Team is funding the study and is also a good partner for discussion. Benedicte Ingstad, Jo Kittelsen, Øyvin Palm, Willy Pedersen, Annick Prieur, Anne Solberg and Kitty Strand have made valuable comments. Jo Kittelsen conducted one of the focus group discussions.

Notes

1   I use the term participant to describe the young men taking part in the project since this phrase best reflects the way their contribution to the project, through spending time and sharing their experiences and emotions.

2   This does not imply that the longing or wish for love does not continue to be just as strong both in this and later periods of life.

References

ABELSON, R.P. (1981) 'Psychological status of the script concept', *American Psychologist,* **36**, 7, pp. 715–29.

COLEMAN, E. (1982) 'Developmental stages of the coming-out process', in P. WILLIAM, J.D. WEINRICH, J.C. GONSIOREK and M.E. HOTVEDT (Eds) *Homosexuality: Social, Psychological and Biological Issues,* London, Sage.

DAVIES, P.M. and WEATHERBURN, P. (1990) 'Towards a general model of sexual negotiation', in P. AGGLETON, G. HART and P. DAVIES (Eds) *AIDS: Responses, Interventions and Care,* London, Falmer Press.

DAVIES, P.M., HICKSON, F.C.I., WEATHERBURN, P. and HUNT, A.J. (1993) *Sex, Gay Men and AIDS,* London, Falmer Press.

DAVIES, P.M., WEATHERBURN, P., HUNT, A.J., HICKSON, F.C.I., MACMANUS, T.J. and COXON, A.P.M. (1992) 'The sexual behaviour of young gay men in England and Wales', *AIDS Care,* **4**, 3, pp. 259–72.

EKSTRAND, M.L. and COATES, T.L. (1990) 'Maintenance of safer sexual behaviors and predictors of risky sex: the San Francisco men's health study', *American Journal of Public Health,* **80**, 8, pp. 973–7.

GAGNON, J.H. (1990) 'The explicit and implicit use of the scripting perspective in sex research', *Annual Review of Sex Research,* **1**, pp. 1–43.

GAGNON, J.H. and SIMON, W. (1973) *Sexual Conduct: The Social Sources of Human Sexuality,* Chicago, Aldine.

HAYS, R., KEGELES, S.M. and COATES, T.J. (1990) 'High HIV risk-taking among gay men', *AIDS,* **4**, pp. 901–7.

HELSEDIREKTORATET (1986) *Helsedirektørens tiltaksplan for bekjempelse av HIV-epidemien,* Oslo.

HELSEDIREKTORATET (1988) *Handlingsplan for skolering og opplysning om hiv/aids,* Oslo.

HELSEDIREKTORATET (1990) *Helsedirektørens tiltaksplan mot HIV/AIDS-epidemien 1990–1995,* Oslo.

KELLY, J.A., ST LAWRENCE, J.S., BRASFIELD T.L. *et al.* (1990) 'Psychosocial factors that predict AIDS high-risk versus AIDS precautionary behavior', *Journal of Consulting and Clinical Psychology,* **58**, 1, pp. 117–20.

KRAFT, PÅL (1990) 'Seksuell débutalder blant norsk ungdom', *Tidsskrift for Norske Lægeforening,* **110**, 23, pp. 3021–4.

KVALEM, INGELA LUNDIN and TRÆEN, BENTE (1995) 'Seksksuelle motiver blant norske ungdommer', *Nordisk Sexologi,* **13**, 2, 85–92.

LAWS, J.L. and SWARTZ, P. (1981) *Sexual Scripts: The Social Construction of Female Sexuality,* Washington: University Press of America.

LEMB, G.F., HIROZAWA, A.M., GIVERTZ, D., NIERI, G.H., ANDERSON, L., LINDGREN, M.L., JANSEN, R.S. and KATZ, M. (1994) 'Seroprevalence of HIV and risk behaviours among young homosexual and bisexual men. The San Francisco/Berkley Young Men's survey', *Journal of the American Medical Association,* **272**, 6, pp. 449–54.

MIDDELTHON, A.L. (1992) 'De Farlige Andre, Om anti-struktur og metaforiserings- og metonymiseringsprosesser i hiv-epidemien', Thesis in Socialanthropology, Oslo: University Oslo.

MIDDELTHON, A.L. (1996) Symbolic Meanings of Condoms Among Young Gay Men in Norway. Poster presented at the XI International Conference on AIDS, Vancouver.

NILSEN, Ø. (1996) National Institute of Public Health, personal communication, Oslo.

PEDERSEN, W., CLAUSEN, S.E. and LAVIK, N.J. (1990) 'Seksuell début: Utviklingen de siste femten årene', *Nordisk Sexologi*, **9**, 3, pp. 194–201.

PLUMMER, K. (1975) *Sexual Stigma: an Interactionist Account*, London, Routledge & Kegan Paul.

PRIEUR, A. (1988) *Kjærlighet mellom menn i aidsens tid*, Oslo: Pax Forlag.

ROTHERAM-BORUS, M.J., HUNTER, J. and ROSARIO, M. (1994) 'Coming out as lesbian or gay in the era of AIDS', in G.M. HEREK and B. GREENE (Eds) *AIDS: Identity, and Community*, London, Sage.

STALL, R. (1992) 'A comparison of younger and older gay men's HIV risk-taking behaviour', *Journal of Acquired Immunodeficiency Syndrome*, **5**, 7, 692–7.

SIMON, W. and GAGNON, J.H. (1986) 'Sexual scripts: permanence and change', *Archives of Sexual Behavior*, **15**, 2, pp. 97–120.

SIMON, W. and GAGNON, J.H. (1987) 'A sexual script's approach', in J.H. GEER and W.T. O'DONOHUE (Eds) *Theories of Human Sexuality*, New York: Plenum Press.

WEATHERBURN, P., HUNT, A.J., HICKSON, F.C.I. and DAVIES, P. (1992) *The Sexual Lifestyles of Gay and Bisexual Men in England and Wales*, London: Project SIGMA.

Chapter 9

HIV Services for Women in East London: The Match between Provision and Needs

Rayah Feldman and Colm Crowley

Professional discourses around care for people living with HIV/AIDS derive from several sources, most notably the tradition of self-help incorporated into the framework of community care (Berridge and Strong, 1991; Feldman, 1994; Weeks, Taylor-Laybourn and Aggleton, 1994). It has often been remarked that in Britain and some other countries, the early impact of AIDS on gay men led to the development of services appropriate to certain kinds of men, and certain kinds of lifestyles, but initially failed to cater for other groups (Berridge and Strong, 1991; Bury, Morrison and McLachlan, 1992; DOH/SSI 1994; Positively Women, 1994). As HIV has spread, so services for other groups have developed but service providers are often unclear about what they should really be offering (Bairstow, 1994). So in social care there is the question of what services to prioritize, for instance, lunch-time drop-ins versus childcare support, counselling versus housing provision. Such decisions involve an understanding of how people cope with living with HIV/AIDS. Both social and medical care also raise the questions of where and how services are delivered, and of eligibility criteria.

This chapter reports on a study of the availability and appropriateness of service provision to women living with HIV in East London. Our broad aim was to explore women's experience of medical and social HIV services within the context of their lives as a whole, as well as to investigate more conventionally how far identifiable services were available and accessible to them. We have extrapolated 'needs' from an understanding of the lives and aspirations of the women we studied. From discussions and interviews with them, it seemed that their 'discourses' around need were in some important respects different from those of service providers and related professionals.

For the women affected, the major life task was to cope with *living with the virus*. To this end they developed a number of coping or 'normalization' strategies.[1] Many women stated explicitly that they 'just wanted to get on' with their lives. Others described the complex stratagems they used to maintain what they perceived as 'normal life'. Now that people are surviving longer after an HIV-positive diagnosis, maintaining normality in one's everyday life can contribute to good health. What differentiates HIV and AIDS services from others is not just the stigma and relative novelty of the illness, but also the diversity of those affected and, increasingly, the recognition that services are about living with HIV infection, possibly for a long time.

Many of the concerns expressed through women's normalization strategies overlap with those of health and social care professionals – and indeed with community care provision. The care demands of HIV/AIDS include community care: can a home be adequately adapted, is there enough home care, is the service user getting the benefits to which they are entitled? These are the rights or entitlements of all sick and disabled people under existing legislation (NHS and Community Care Act, 1990; DOH, 1993). It *is* important to investigate whether these are being recognized and provided, and where the bottlenecks and inadequacies are in their provision. Doing this has been a major part of our research but such investigation also throws up much ambiguity and confusion about how community care should contribute towards living an ordinary life as opposed to a narrower conception of managing disease.

Many specialist HIV services are justly regarded as innovatory and excellent. All the women who got help from statutory agencies and voluntary sector organizations found many of the services and the individuals who offered them helpful, despite frequent dissatisfaction with particular services. Our aim here is to highlight aspects of services that merit critical attention and to identify areas where improvements could be made, while acknowledging the quality of many services.

Women have been studied primarily in relation to their reproductive role rather than in terms of their own health and wellbeing (Henderson, 1992; Scharf, 1992). Attention to women is important not only in its own right, as increasing numbers of women become affected by HIV. It also has the advantage of enabling us to broaden our view of the impact of the epidemic on all people's lives. In particular, studying women highlights the impact of HIV on children and the family, which has been a relatively neglected area in HIV research so far (except in relation to counselling). However, it is important to recognize that men have families too and even look after children of their own or children left to their care (Cates *et al.*, 1990; Honigsbaum, 1991; Powell, 1992; Spurrier, 1994).

A focus on women also draws attention to the issue of gender: how women's roles and social situations differ from men's; how women are treated both publicly and privately, and hence how HIV affects women's lives in different ways from men's and how it affects the relationships between men and women. At the same time women affected by HIV also differ from each other and share many of the same social and medical problems as men. They are often and even typically bound up in a range of intimate personal relationships with men who are themselves affected by HIV.

So in looking at the relationship between service provision and the needs of women, we have found ourselves having to address a lack of clarity both in the way community care services have been conceptualized and in the way practitioners and commentators think about women and women's service needs. Community care appears to have been designed as a 'moveable feast', in that the legislation is deliberately vague and provides few specific entitlements to clients (Rao, 1991; Baldwin, 1993; Walker, 1993). But at the same time, its very vagueness provides scope for creativity. The directions for that creativity are being and will be forged by struggles to articulate and legitimize new needs of a wide range of people facing hitherto unpredicted situations. Gay men in particular have already been hugely influential in challenging traditional forms of service provision for the disabled and chronically sick and condemning them as inappropriate for them in facing AIDS. They have also reaffirmed their social solidarity in inventing and establishing new forms of provision. The scope for similar challenges by very diverse groups of women still remains. We hope this chapter can contribute to this task.

Methods

The study was restricted to women affected by HIV in four East London boroughs. The main source of information for the study came from taped, in-depth, semi-structured interviews with 37 women, of whom 28 were HIV-positive, and 9 were living in close relationships with infected individuals, or were the bereaved relatives of people who had had HIV disease. Their ages ranged from 21 to 50. Nine respondents were British, 22 were African, and the remainder were from Ireland, continental Europe and North America. Thirty-one were currently living in East London or had lived there at the time of diagnosis. Six respondents lived elsewhere in London but used voluntary sector HIV services in at least one of the four boroughs.

In common with many studies of this kind, accessing respondents and getting their agreement to be interviewed was very difficult, partly because of confidentiality, and partly because many service users and professionals felt that they were already giving information to numerous researchers, ostensibly for policy purposes, with no noticeable effect on services. While the problem of over-research and policy implementation was beyond our control, we found that group discussions had particular merits. First, they helped people feel their voice was being heard. Second, women seemed more willing to come with friends to a group, especially if it was linked to a meal and if childcare was provided, than to an individual interview with a stranger. Third, different kinds of issues are raised in groups. The experience of discussion helps people to reflect on their experience, rather than merely describe it. Finally, a good discussion group generated trust, so that many women agreed to individual interviews *after* they had participated in a group.

We held three focus groups with different women. The first group consisted of twelve women, eleven of whom were HIV-positive. The twelfth woman was the mother of one of the participants. Another group consisted of three women, of whom two were HIV-positive and the third was the wife and carer of an HIV-positive man. The third group comprised ten HIV-positive women and three professionals whom most of the women knew well. This group provided an opportunity for us to observe an interchange between the professionals and the service users. The gap between their discourses, despite much mutual trust and respect, was the inspiration behind this paper.

Other methods of obtaining information included participant observation in voluntary organizations and at meetings. Discussions or more formal, semi-structured interviews were held with more than 30 workers from both the statutory and voluntary sectors in each borough, including social services professionals, community nurse specialists, health advisors and representatives of nearly all relevant local HIV voluntary organizations.

Using this multiplicity of methods we managed to obtain a picture of a wide range of women both in terms of transmission route and social and domestic circumstances. Although the women we met were not terminally ill, several women had had serious bouts of illness and at least one woman has died since being interviewed. Several of the HIV-positive women we saw had not been diagnosed as having AIDS .

In the interviews we tracked women's lives from the time they were affected by HIV. From this we have tried to identify the needs that they expressed either explicitly or implicity. We met some of the women we interviewed several times and were able to get to know them. In the discussion groups we were also able to gather information about women whom we did not interview individually. The interviews with professionals informed us how they saw the services and their perceptions of the problems of service provision for women.

Race, Culture, HIV and Inner Cities

Our study was conducted in four adjacent boroughs: Hackney, Newham, Tower Hamlets and Waltham Forest. This is an area characterized by a high reported prevalence of HIV and particularly high reported rates of HIV infection among women. Indeed, Newham has the highest reported rate of HIV infection among women outside Lothian in Scotland. Estimates of numbers infected and affected are difficult to obtain, but Table 9.1 shows the reported number of HIV infected men and women in these boroughs.

The boroughs themselves are typical of inner-London boroughs, with high rates of poverty and unemployment. Historically, they have also been the destination of new immigrants and refugees. The racialized connotation

Table 9.1 *Women in East London with an HIV Diagnosis (1994 Figures)* *

Probable transmission route	Hackney	Newham	Tower Hamlets	Waltham Forest and Redbridge
Women – probably heterosex. acquired infection	16	61	17	26
Women – probably injecting drug use	8	2	3	3
All reported diagnosed infections (men/women)	202	247	219	221

* These figures exclude women probably infected by other routes, and are also likely to be a slight underestimate of the true figure because of under-reporting or failure of the cases reported to fulfil the qualifying criteria for inclusion in the statistics. Under-reporting is likely to have less effect on the numbers of women than men. (Personal communication, J. O'Sullivan, East London and City Health Authority)
Source: *HIV Information Exchange*: coordinated by the Public Health Laboratory Service, Communicable Diseases Surveillance Centre.

in British political discourse of the term 'immigrants' has, since the 1950s, given the impression that all immigrants are poor, Black and unskilled, hence also uneducated, rootless and dangerous. As a result, open discussion on the specific problems of HIV and minority communities has to some extent been stifled to avoid inflaming racism further (Bhatt, 1995).

A second response, particularly characteristic of social work and, in our view, just as damaging, has been to designate immigrants and Black people generally as victims of circumstance, of racism and often patronizingly, of 'culture'. The effects of culture are simply alluded to in often vague and un-specific ways. For example, Barlow claims that 'many women from minority backgrounds will be affected by religious and social proscriptions, due to certain fundamentalist traditions within their own cultures or tribal customs' (Barlow, 1992, p. 27). She claims that as a result 'women from sub-Saharan Africa tend to present very late for help at services in London', but offers no explanation of what such traditions or customs are and how they produce this effect.

Recent concerns about 'cultural sensitivity', while well-intentioned, tend to reify culture and to regard it as a fixed property nearly always attached to 'other' people. Such approaches ignore the cultural preconceptions within which professional disciplines and organizations themselves operate. They also tend to see other people's culture, at best, as something to be sensitive to and, at worst, as a barrier to rational behaviour. For instance, we have fre-quently heard professionals attribute to 'culture' the failure of HIV-affected women to make complaints, to question professionals, to know about or to use services. This conception of culture overlays many professionals' view of, especially, African service users, and prevents them being seen as women with education, experience, skills and strategies for survival. It also provides a ready 'explanation' of service deficiencies without requiring reflexivity or self-examination.

Types of Deficiencies in Services

Inadequacies in HIV services have as much to do with a failure to recognize and acknowledge how women have to deal with HIV/AIDS in the context of their whole lives as with straightforward resource constraints. We have identified several kinds of deficiencies in services in this study, all of which may exist in any kind of social and health provision. While the effects of some of them are self-evident, especially where services fall short of basic standards, we are looking at them specifically in terms of their negative impact on people's capacity to live 'normally' with HIV/AIDS.

Sub-standard Services

Sub-standard services are those which fall below acceptable standards because of poor quality, delays or insufficent provision. Examples cited by respondents in this study include poor quality housing, delays in getting benefits, long waits in out-patient clinics or too little homecare. Service users also experienced breaches of confidentiality in hospital departments not specializing in HIV-related care, where the use of special stickers on blood samples or distinctive notices on doors publicly identified them as HIV-positive (Henderson, 1991; Positively Women, 1994).

Inappropriate Service Standards

Inappropriate service standards mean that services do not achieve their intended objectives for clients. Services have often developed in particular ways because of mistaken assumptions about service users, or because they are geared to a specific client group. This may have the effect that although services are technically available they are still not accessible to users. For example, HIV-related clinics in hospitals often make no childcare provision because they have been designed for men with no childcare responsibilities.

This is so in spite of the many innovations that characterize such clinics compared with hospital services for other conditions. On the other hand, social service children's services have developed in response to statutory child protection concerns rather than to provide flexible childcare support for chronically sick women. Similarly, most medical and social service appointments, and even complementary therapies and support groups for people living with HIV/AIDS, take place in working hours and cannot be used by people with regular jobs.

In some cases inappropriate standards stem from services having been designed to suit the convenience of providers rather than users. Common complaints related to service users having to cope with frequent changes of professional staff and a general lack of communication between professionals and service users. To change professional staff without informing patients or clients is a practice that is relatively common in the health service and common in social services, but one which ignores the impact on service users. Women in one focus group also complained vociferously that inexplicably large numbers of blood samples were taken from them in hospital with no attempt to explain why they were needed.

Lack of Information

The community care system itself as a model of provision based on consumer choice is very dependent on adequate communications' systems. The diversity of services and providers which is supposed to enhance such choice is of little use if service users are not told about them. Yet systems of communicating information are *ad hoc* and depend very much on prior connections.

Until now gay men have been best placed to know and pass on information about HIV services because of their place in the history of the epidemic and the degree of self-organization and openness which the gay community developed in response to HIV and AIDS. Many gay men are also prominent figures in AIDS service organizations. Other people affected by HIV, including many women, are much more isolated from HIV-related networks and are hence much more dependant on formal channels of information about services and their entitlements to them. Our research suggests that organizations and health and social services professionals are important sources of information, but that unless people are in regular contact with an agency they are unlikely to be well-informed about services. There is no systematic mechanism within the social or healthcare system to check and review on a regular basis whether information relevant to clients' current situation and state of health has been made available to them. As a result, and as people's circumstances and needs change, they are often not aware either that certain services are available or how to access them.

Inappropriate Criteria of Eligibility

People are often excluded from services and benefits because they are asymptomatic though HIV-positive. Two important attributes of HIV infection call for a modification of traditional conceptions of the appropriate moment or threshold for entitlement to social care, whether this be benefits, improved housing or childcare services. First, the nature of HIV disease and the rapidly changing methods of managing it mean that people with HIV may be wholly asymptomatic either for a long period before any symptoms are manifested, or they may have intermittent periods of no or mild symptoms. Second, the stigma of HIV and its probably fatal outcome mean that an HIV diagnosis alone generates anxiety and stress for the person diagnosed and their immediate family beyond that experienced in other, even fatal diseases. Stigma significantly constrains people's capacity to lead 'normal' lives and this itself generates stress. It is increasingly acknowledged by health practitioners with experience of HIV that stress itself creates symptoms of ill-health and may reduce a person's capacity to resist and deal with opportunistic infections (Leonard and Miller, 1995).

Childcare services, for example, may be crucial in reducing stress and overwork, particularly for parents (and usually mothers), helping them stay well and sustain the family unit longer. In this sense, the provision of family services to asymptomatic HIV-positive adults may even be seen as a cost-effective form of service provision. However, children's services are often thought necessary only if the child is infected or the mother is seriously ill. Similarly, good housing, or certain disability benefits, provided even if the beneficiaries are asymptomatic, could contribute to the longer-term maintenance of good health. As it is, services and benefits available to asymptomatic HIV infected people are somewhat arbitrary and tend to be very limited.

Absence of Services

HIV has generated or added weight to demands for new kinds of services such as complementary therapies, social support or the provision of high quality cooked food. One study has compared HIV to a barium meal which shows up the defective parts of housing associations (Yates, 1989). It highlights similar blockages in the community care system. It also exposes gaps in our understanding of the kind of support people need to continue to live normally with a chronic disease. Women living with HIV/AIDS are a relatively new client group with new needs and new problems of policy implementation. 'Family support', a relatively new concept in social work, which has been developed largely to prevent family crisis, may provide a framework for new types of children's and family services which will meet the new kinds of needs that living with HIV creates (Donnelly, 1993). HIV also creates particular problems for people in maintaining social relationships which call for innovative solutions. Labelling individual or social problems as health or social care 'needs' can be contentious but is essential if services are really intended to help people *live* with chronic illness.

It is not always easy to classify concrete experiences of deficiencies in services within a single category. What is common to many of them is a failure of services to respond to the long-term nature of HIV disease and how it is embedded in people's daily lives. Many people living with HIV/AIDS have other problems in their lives that HIV services cannot solve, but HIV can exacerbate any one of them. For example, one woman had a violent partner who had threatened to kill her if he found she was HIV-positive. Several women were asylum-seekers without refugee status. As such they were unable to bring other children or their parents to join them, but because of their HIV diagnosis they had long-term anxieties over what would happen to children overseas when they themselves died. The two women in regular employment found that HIV affected many aspects of their working lives, including their job security, sickness absences or stress from working long hours.

Support for women living with HIV must take these kinds of issues into account in service design, recognizing how immediate pressures on such women may be linked to wider problems or longer-term strategies to remain in control of or to 'normalize' their lives. In particular, people can make adjustments best when they are well, yet most services are activated only when they are sick.

Problems of 'Normalization'

Visibility

One response of AIDS professionals to the stigma of HIV has been to increase their vigilance about maintaining confidentiality in order to prevent the identification of service users as HIV-positive. This has sometimes gone to counterproductive lengths as when information on service users is not shared between professionals. Yet from the viewpoint of the service user the issue of confidentiality may be as much about 'visibility' or being conspicuous within the broader social world as about what is disclosed about her between professionals.

Within debates on HIV, justifications for the importance of maintaining confidentiality have been given largely in rationalist terms: how an HIV-positive diagnosis affects a person's job security, access to mortgages or insurance, for example. Confidentiality, however, is also important in relation to how people are seen and treated as they conduct their everyday life. There is a danger that the welfare system around HIV confers a badge of identity. For the service user the problem is how to accept the services without the badge. This can be illustrated by the following examples.

Some African women described how uncomfortable they feel when taking holidays at dedicated HIV centres in Bournemouth and Cornwall. This is because, as African women in very 'white' areas, they can be identified as 'coming from the HIV centre' when they visit the town or village nearby. One woman contrasted this with a holiday in a bed-and-breakfast in the Isle of Wight organized by an HIV women's group, where they posed as a 'Keep Fit' group on a weekend away and had a much more relaxed time.

Women identified similar problems of visibility when using taxi-cards and disabled travel passes. Several women reported being viewed with suspicion by bus drivers and other passengers who evidently thought they were fraudsters when using their disabled passes. They perceived them as thinking, 'What is a well-dressed woman doing with a free bus pass?' They are also worried that taxi drivers contracted by agencies know their destination and why they are travelling on account. Some women say they prefer to make their own arrangements and then get reimbursed.

Similar concerns troubled one woman in relation to people recognizing the standard issue furniture in her housing association flat. Another woman did not want to use a grant because people would wonder where a woman receiving income support got a new washing-machine from. A non-HIV-positive woman whose husband had AIDS worried about what neighbours would say about a childless couple being allocated a two-bedroom flat.

Visibility is obviously a difficult issue to resolve. While service providers may recognize the importance of providing practical services for people living with HIV/AIDS, they need to take into account how it is provided in order to preserve service users' anonymity and reduce unwelcome conspicuousness.

Employment

Only three of the women we talked with were in full-time work. Other women have worked sporadically. There seems to be an overall assumption in AIDS service organizations that women service users are *not* in work. This is partly linked to assumptions that women's HIV services are always linked with children. Women are often not visible to service providers except as mothers. As a result, services for women without children, and especially for women in work, are notably absent. Such women find hospital appointments, complementary therapies and support groups difficult to access.

Daytime appointments are particularly problematic for service users in work as they find it difficult to keep negotiating sick leave without disclosing their HIV status. One woman was worried that repeated sickness absences for hospital appointments and to cover monthly plasma donation gave the impression that she was ill, when in fact she enjoyed very good health. She was concerned that her sickness record would affect future job prospects. However, to disclose her HIV status in her present temporary job by explaining these absences might prevent her contract being renewed.

Another effect of assuming that women living with HIV/AIDS are not working, results in the absence of any support to enable service users, including carers, to re-enter employment. Yet being HIV-positive, or living with someone who is, does not make a person unemployable. While obviously if someone is very sick, paid work may become difficult, until such a time, work provides income and self-esteem. Moreover, work does not have to be full-time. 'Flexible work' does not need to be simply a codename for casual work, but is also a concept that is being developed as part of equal opportunities (*New Ways to Work Newsletter*, 1995).

Many women living with HIV are very well educated and potentially employable. Though figures are small and must be treated with caution, a 10 per cent sample study from the 1991 Census shows that Black Africans are the second most highly qualified ethnic group in Newham, with 17.3 per cent qualified, exceeded only by the Chinese, with 20.83 per cent qualified (Office of Population Censuses and Surveys, 1993, Table 9). Many African immigrants have been in professional employment in their own countries, and most of the women we met were English-speaking and would have no difficulty coping with jobs. More than half the women from all backgrounds whom we interviewed were college educated (17 out of 31 for whom we have this information).

Support for women living with HIV/AIDS to return to study or to specific training would be especially useful for people who have been educated and have developed skills overseas, and whose qualifications and experience may not be recognized in the UK. Several women in the study have, in fact, enrolled on further and higher education courses when they could get childcare support, but such support is also subject to the constraints of eligibility discussed earlier. It is not fanciful to envisage the development of career advice for people living with HIV/AIDS as part of a strategy to help them normalize their lives.

Isolation

Isolation is frequently cited as a problem both for HIV-positive women and for women carers. Support groups have developed partly in response to this problem and many women find them of enormous benefit. But they cannot solve all the problems of isolation or its effects. Here we discuss two little considered aspects of isolation.

Telephones

Telephones were often referred to in the individual and group discussions with women. Almost all women from overseas reported having had their telephones cut off at different times, and there seems to be no uniformity between authorities in the policy on payment of telephone bills or rental. Yet telephones function to keep people in touch, especially if they are unwell and poor. African women used telephones a lot partly to maintain important family contacts at home – with elderly parents or with children left behind who have no right of entry into the UK. Many of the women now in England continue to play an important part in managing family affairs at home. In some cases they use the telephone to trace missing relatives lost in war zones.

Many professionals recognized the problem of telephone disconnection and high bills but were able to offer little practical assistance. Some boroughs paid telephone rental charges but no more. Some women had received help with telephone bills from voluntary organizations. One social worker felt that the issue was just one of money management and thought that people should be taught to budget and needed to be trained to be independent. Our view is that budgeting, although important, is not really the issue. Having no telephone can increase the need for other forms of care. One woman complained that she did not have enough homecare given that she was not well and was not on the telephone as it had been disconnected. Her social worker responded that she was not eligible for more homecare, in terms of her health, but she knew no way to get the telephone reinstated as there was an outstanding debt. Yet without a telephone this woman remains isolated, liable to depression and more vulnerable to deteriorating health. Telephones could be seen as a cost-effective contribution to social care in much the same way as taxi-cards and free travel passes.

Carers

Within families, the carer role is particularly gendered. Women typically have the job of managing emotional situations in families and they also often have to care directly for the HIV-positive person. Nevertheless, the question of support for carers is insufficiently addressed by providers – their job is to *give* support rather than *get* it (Miller, 1987; Tavanyar, 1992; Hull-York, 1993; Warwick, 1993). One woman described how she felt trapped by guilt into not challenging the unacceptable behaviour of her dying son for whom she was caring. She was helped to deal with her son's behaviour by the HIV-specialist nurse who was visiting regularly because of her son's condition. Had her son been less ill and not receiving these visits she would have been without support. Carers or partners of less-sick patients may lack such professional support

because they have less contact with services. However, even with good support from health or social services, they often remain socially isolated. This
is particularly true if the carers are themselves HIV-positive (Henderson, 1991;
Watney, 1993). One woman we met was herself HIV-positive, and supported
herself and her very sick husband by working long hours in a professional job
which involved dealing with other people's problems. She found the strain
very hard to bear.

Women carers can experience particular isolation because of the pressures
of caring and being housebound. HIV-negative carers are also not eligible
for many HIV services targeted to women which are restricted to women who
are HIV-positive. Yet the chronic, long-term and fluctuating nature of HIV
infection creates distinctive pressures, and may mean that the carer will live
in a situation of stress, stigma, isolation and unpredictability for many years.
She may be playing a key role in nursing or more generally in maintaining
the health of the person she is caring for. In one borough, service providers'
concern to preserve confidentiality prevented them from putting women carers
in touch with each other, even though one carer very much wanted to meet
other women in the same situation as herself.

Sexual Relationships and Marriage

Women in marriages and other long-term relationships face different problems
from women outside such relationships. Problems in sexual relationships for
HIV-positive women have been discussed mainly in terms of the general difficulties women have negotiating safer sex rather than in relation to specific
types or patterns of couple relationships (O'Sullivan, 1992; Positively Women,
1994; Green, 1995).

This study showed how power inequalities within heterosexual couples
living with HIV/AIDS are also exacerbated by other circumstances, and can
affect women's ability to access services, look after themselves and meet other
people socially. Relationships with men increased the problems faced by many
of the African women in our study. Male refugees experience different problems of dislocation and loss of position and self-esteem than women. Within
the home they often compensate by either lack of support for, or aggression
towards, their partners. They may manifest excessive alcohol use, domestic
violence and mental health problems, as well as refusal to deal with sexually
transmitted diseases.[2] One service provider said that in her view, the single
most important help to African women would be services for African men.

These kinds of problems seem to be particularly prevalent among refugees, but violence and threats of violence occur among all people and may
often be exacerbated by an HIV or AIDS diagnosis (Basche and Partridge,

1994). Women experiencing domestic violence can find themselves doubly isolated. Domestic violence itself is often accompanied by enforced isolation. Women living with HIV/AIDS may also find themselves less able to access services because of it. One woman we interviewed had been unable to take up hospital appointments because of threatened violence by her partner if he discovered she had AIDS. This was in spite of the fact that he himself manifested many symptoms of HIV infection. We do not know whether women are given information about services like women's refuges by HIV voluntary organizations or social workers, or how far refuge workers are HIV-aware.

Family Life and Childcare

As far as women with children are concerned, maintaining their children's lives without disruption and protecting them from the effects of stigma is possibly the highest priority. Nowhere is the aspiration to lead a 'normal' life clearer than in relation to the care of children and the maintenance of the family. Yet, not only have HIV-specialist services been primarily oriented to adults, but statutory children's and family services have been very slow to consider the needs of HIV-affected families (Donnelly, 1993; Lyon, 1995; Feldman and Ndofor-Tah, 1996).

Such families have very specific needs which relate to both the social and medical aspects of living with HIV. These needs are much more like those facing families with parents or children with other disabilities, and include respite care for children when the caring parent is in hospital, or is too weak or unwell, or giving the parent some time to help reduce stress. As the course of HIV disease is unpredictable, the type of childcare support needed will vary over time. Parents may also need support with long-term planning for their children but often have difficulties in acknowledging this or finding the right time to begin the process.

Families with children require access to flexible, rapid care. This may range from short-term emergency baby-sitting to permanent care. Families receiving palliative care may need carers for their children to come to the family home in order to minimize disruption. The idea of providing care at a client's home is relatively new within family services, but is very appropriate to HIV-affected families and may also be of value to other groups.

The East London Childcare Initiative (ELCI) was set up in 1994 jointly by the boroughs of Hackney, Tower Hamlets, Newham and Waltham Forest, in response to these needs. It has been working since then to develop appropriate, flexible care within mainstream services for children from HIV-affected families. ELCI's work has also raised the issue of providing childcare services to HIV-positive parents who are asymptomatic.

Information

Women in the study expressed a desire for more knowledge about three main aspects of living with HIV/AIDS: medical information, what services were available and how the health and social care system works. Participation in groups has been used as an important means of information-sharing. It was evident from observation, as well as to the women themselves, that better knowledge about how to manage the progression of the disease would give them more control over their lives.

Medical Information

Women were keen to have a range of information both about their own condition and treatments, and especially about transmission risks to babies. This latter concern came especially from African women who also expressed concern about anonymous antenatal testing. While on the one hand there has been concern by professionals that named testing has been disproportionately offered to 'high risk' women, especially African women, the policy of anonymous testing, which is of value to researchers and policy-makers rather than to individual women, does not seem to have been discussed with members of this same 'high risk' group. Several HIV-positive women in the study were, in fact, not tested antenatally, and therefore when they were later diagnosed, they were devastated to learn that they could have taken precautions to reduce the vertical transmission risk, including avoiding breastfeeding.

Our impression from the women in the study is that women in 'high risk' groups want to know if they are HIV-positive because they want to do everything they can to have healthy babies. This view goes against some current orthodoxies (Scharf, 1992) but suggests that health professionals need to consult with women from communities where there is a high prevalence of HIV, about their attitudes to HIV-testing.

Information about Available Services and how the Community Care System Works

Lack of information is perhaps the most frustrating element in community care. It is hard to separate lack of knowledge of which services are available from lack of knowledge about how the system works. Since few people seem to understand the arcane logic of the community care system, for service users the important issue is to know which services are available and how to access them. Some women make it a lifetime's study; others have no idea what is available. At first sight, women's ability to access services is like a lottery. On closer inspection, it is clear that women who have contacts with supportive professionals often acquire information directly, and are also thereby helped to develop the confidence to attend groups where information is informally shared. However, few women had participated in groups whose *formal* purpose was the dissemination and exchange of information. Yet our own focus groups were used by participants as information exchanges both among themselves and between them and the professionals who took part.

A lack of opportunity to find out how the community care system works, even its variability and apparent arbitrariness, is very disempowering for many service users. It also prevents complaints. It has been suggested that 'it is a culturally unfamiliar concept to formally complain in many societies' (Local Authority Associations' Working Group on AIDS, 1995, p. 23). However, until the present government elevated the principle of complaint to the equivalent of consumer sovereignty, formal complaints were unfamiliar here, too. African women do not complain for the same reasons as other people: in some cases they feel that it would be against their interests to rock the boat; in other cases they lack information about procedures and do not know where to direct a complaint. Failure to complain is not caused by cultural barriers but by practical ones.

Several women complained in a group discussion about what they felt was the excessive collection of blood samples. When asked why they had not complained at the time, they said that once they had asked why so much blood was needed, and got unsatisfactory replies, they acquiesced, not wanting to be seen as 'bad' patients and knowing that they had to maintain an ongoing relationship with the medical staff. Another reason people do not complain is because of their unfamiliarity with the system. One woman who suspected serious medical negligence said that in her country she would have sued, but here she did not know whom to contact or how to go about it.

Improved information flows, and opportunities to have one's voice heard, especially in a group where one can have a dialogue with professionals, would often obviate the need for complaints. It would also provide feedback to providers, and hopefully give both providers and service users a better understanding of each other's respective concerns and priorities. The power that knowledge of one's medical condition, of treatments and of the care system itself, confers, is not to displace professionals, but rather to be able to take more control of one's own life.

Implications for Services

Our characterization of living with HIV/AIDS as involving aspirations to 'normalize' life as far as possible calls for a reappraisal of the goals of HIV services. We suggest that such services need consider not only helping people to manage the *disease* as it progresses, but also to manage many *other* aspects of their lives – when people diagnosed HIV-positive are well, as well as when they are sick.

Heightened concern with confidentiality has been a distinguishing feature of HIV services and professional attitudes and has almost come to be a shibboleth of the HIV world. However, professionals' focus on stratagems to preserve clients' confidentiality *within* HIV services may have been at the expense of seeing the problem of confidentiality in a wider context. The specialization of HIV services in response to pressure from affected people, mainly gay men, and to the AIDS Support Grant, has resulted in some splendid and innovative services. As the range of affected people widens, especially to include more women and children from ethnic-minority communities, such services may nevertheless exclude potentially eligible clients whose needs these services fail to address. The AIDS-affected community needs to find ways of developing services within the mainstream which are accessible and appropriate to a wider range of people, but which do not lose some of the innovative features of earlier HIV projects. The East London Childcare Initiative is an example of a movement in that direction. Such developments also require consultation with the people whose needs they are trying to address – and imaginative ways of reaching them may be necessary.

Finally, we have pinpointed the problem of reconciling choice with lack of information within the new community care system. We have been struck by the haphazard flow of information about services to clients, and a lack of systems of feedback to professionals. Improving information flows to service users should be a continuing process in order to meet different needs at different times. Above all, initial contact must be made and then sustained between professionals and service users. This may involve outreach work followed by a system of mentoring in which service users have a single professional from whom they can get information and support. A mentor acting as informant and advocate can help service users access both individual and group services.

An inter-agency, inter-borough, regularly updated handbook would reduce the need for the duplication of information within boroughs and agencies and could be routinely given out to service users. Much information is inevitably acquired informally through social interaction, but facilitating participation in HIV settings takes a long time and participation may not be possible for everyone. Information and training sessions for service users about the different aspects of living with HIV/AIDS can also be used as opportunities for feedback to professionals about service user concerns.

Community care, for all its defects, has considerable potential in providing a range of services for people living with a chronic illness such as HIV/AIDS. The dissemination of information is crucial if this potential is to be realized.

Notes

1   Gorna's (1996) characterization of AIDS as 'queer in the sense of not normal' adds power and poignancy to the argument made here that women affected by HIV and AIDS want to normalize their lives.

2   We do not have evidence for this other than reports from respondents, supported by in-depth interviews with an HIV professional with strong roots in the Ugandan refugee community, a Ugandan pastor and discussions with other Ugandan refugees. 'Traditional' male supremacist attitudes which are also held responsible for difficulties which African women face (Ama Amamoo, 1996) are likely to be strengthened in the adverse circumstances in which many refugees find themselves.

References

AMA AMAMOO, N. (1996) *Working with Men for Change: Gender and HIV Prevention in the African Community in the UK*, London: Akina Mama wa Afrika.

BAIRSTOW, S. (1994) 'The social worker's role', in L. CUSACK and S. SINGH (Eds) *HIV and AIDS Care: Practical Approaches*, London: Chapman & Hall.

BALDWIN, S. (1993) *The Myth of Community Care*, London: Chapman & Hall.

BARLOW, J. (1992) 'Social issues: an overview', in J. BURY, V. MORRISON and S. MCLACHLAN (Eds) *Working with Women and AIDS: Medical, Social and Counselling Issues*, London: Routledge.

BASCHE, M. and PARTRIDGE, J. (1994) 'Domestic violence against HIV-positive women', paper presented at the 2nd Biopsychosocial Aspects of HIV Infection Conference, Brighton.

BERRIDGE, V. and STRONG, P. (1991) 'AIDS in the UK: contemporary history and social policy', *Twentieth Century British History*, **2**, 2, pp. 150–74.

BHATT, C. (1995) *Needs Assessment for HIV Prevention – HIV and Black Communities 3*, London: The HIV Project.

BURY, J., MORRISON, V. and MCLACHLAN, S. (1992) *Working with Women and AIDS: Medical, Social and Counselling Issues*, London: Routledge.

CATES, J.A., GRAHAM, L., BOEGLIN, D. and TIELKER, S. (1990) 'The effect of AIDS on the family system', *Families in Society*, **71**, 3, pp. 195–201.

DEPARTMENT OF HEALTH (1993) *Implementing Caring for People: Community Care for People with HIV and AIDS*, London: Department of Health.

DEPARTMENT OF HEALTH/SOCIAL SERVICES INSPECTORATE (1994) *Women and HIV*, London: Department of Health.

DONNELLY, D. (1993) *Have We Got it Right?* HIV/AIDS Children's Research Project, London: Hammersmith and Fulham Council.

FELDMAN, R. (1994) 'User empowerment: contradictions between self-help and service delivery in AIDS service voluntary organisations', unpublished paper presented at *AIDS Impact*, the 2nd International Conference on Biopsychosocial Aspects of HIV Infection, Brighton.

FELDMAN, R. and NDOFOR-TAH, C. (1996) 'The East London Child Care Initiative – Activities and Impact 1994–6' (Unpublished Report to the North Thames Regional Health Authority).

GORNA, R. (1996) *Vamps, Virgins and Victims – How Can Women Fight AIDS?* London: Cassell.

GREEN, G. (1995) 'Sex, love and seropositivity: balancing the risks', in P. AGGLETON, P. DAVIES and G. HART (Eds) *AIDS: Safety, Sexuality and Risk*, London: Taylor & Francis.

HENDERSON, S. (1991) 'Care: what's in it for her?', in P. AGGLETON, G. HART and P. DAVIES (Eds) *AIDS: Responses, Interventions and Care*, London: Falmer Press.

HENDERSON, S. (1992) 'Living with the virus: perspectives from HIV positive women in London', in N. DORN, S. HENDERSON and N. SOUTH (Eds) *AIDS: Women, Drugs and Social Care*, London: Falmer Press.

HONIGSBAUM, N. (1991) *HIV, AIDS and Children: A Cause for Concern*, London: National Children's Bureau.

HULL–YORK RESEARCH TEAM (1993) *Social Care and HIV/AIDS*, London: HMSO.

LEONARD, B. and MILLER, K. (1995) *Stress, the Immune System and Psychiatry*, Chichester: John Wiley.

LOCAL AUTHORITY ASSOCIATIONS' OFFICER WORKING GROUP ON AIDS (LAAWGA) (1995) *Learning from African Families*, London: The Local Government Management Board.

LYON, J. (1995) *Newham Social Services – Children and Families and HIV/AIDS*, London: Jennifer Lyon Research.

MILLER, D. (1987) *Living with AIDS and HIV*, Basingstoke: Macmillan.

New Ways to Work Newsletter (1995) London: New Ways to Work.

NHS AND COMMUNITY CARE ACT (1990) London: HMSO.

OFFICE OF POPULATION CENSUSES AND SURVEYS (OPCS) (1993) *1991 Census: County Report for Inner London (Part 2)*, London: HMSO.

O'SULLIVAN, S. (1992) 'Sex in difficult times', in S. O'SULLIVAN and K. THOMSON (Eds) *Positively Women*, London, Sheba.

POSITIVELY WOMEN (1994) *Women Like Us*, London: Positively Women.

POWELL, P. (1992) *Meeting the Challenge of HIV/AIDS in Women and Children*, Norwich: Social Work Monographs.

RAO, N. (1991) *From Providing to Enabling: Local Authorities qnd Community Care Planning*, York: Joseph Rowntree Foundation.

SCHARF, E. (1992) 'Research: HIV/AIDS and the Invisibility of Women', in S. O'SULLIVAN and K. THOMSON (Eds) *Positively Women: Living with AIDS*, London: Sheba.

SPURRIER, L. (1994) *AIDS in the Family*, London: Hodder & Stoughton.

TAVANYAR, J. (1992) *The Terrence Higgins Trust HIV/AIDS Book*, London: Thorsons.

WALKER, A. (1993) 'Community care policy: from consensus to conflict', in J. BORNAT,

C. PEREIRA, D. PILGRIM and F. WILLIAMS (Eds) *Community Care: a Reader*, London: Macmillan in association with the Open University Press.

WARWICK, I. (1993) 'Exploring informal sector care: the need for assessed, evaluated and resourced support', in P. AGGLETON, P. DAVIES and G. HART (Eds) *AIDS: Facing the Second Decade*, London: Falmer Press.

WATNEY, S. (1993) 'AIDS: the second decade: "risk", research and modernity', in P. AGGLETON, G. HART and P. DAVIES (Eds) *AIDS: Responses, Interventions and Care*, London: Falmer Press.

WEEKS, J., TAYLOR-LAYBOURN, A. and AGGLETON, P. (1994) 'An anatomy of the HIV/AIDS voluntary sector in Britain', in P. AGGLETON and G. HART (Eds) *AIDS: Foundations for the Future*, London: Taylor & Francis.

YATES, C. (1989) *Housing and HIV Disease*, London: National Federation of Housing Associations.

Chapter 10

Professionalism and Sexual Identity in Gay and Bisexual Men's HIV Prevention

Katie Deverell

This chapter is based on material collected while examining how HIV-prevention outreach workers construct personal and professional boundaries within work, and between work and other parts of their lives. The research is specifically focused on sexual boundaries and gay and bisexual men's HIV-prevention activities. Most of the information has been collected through in-depth interviews with gay men, although the research has also included interviews with some bisexual men, lesbians and heterosexual women.[1]

All the workers are paid and involved (to a greater or lesser degree) in outreach work with gay, bisexual and other men who have sex with men. Their jobs are perhaps unusual because their professional concern is defined in relation to sex and sexuality. The work involves, for example, talking about sex; giving condoms, lubricants, advice and information to men in settings where they meet to socialize or have sex; and using techniques, insights and strategies developed from their own sexual experiences. This means that sexuality and sex are a part of work and not something separate to it. The fact that the work is HIV-related also produces an association of sex with work.

Despite this association, many of the workers tried to draw personal and professional boundaries and keep their own sexual life separate from work. This was achieved primarily in relation to not having sex with the men they were working with, not meeting their own sexual needs through work, and by making a space for their own sexual needs to be met.

A constant theme which emerged during the interviews on boundaries was the workers' reference to being professional, and in particular to the relationship between professionalism and sexual identity. This relationship raised many tensions and issues which will be explored in this chapter. As a starting point, the following two quotes are intended to signal some of the different ways in which the relationship of sexual identity and professionalism was seen.

> This one I feel I have difficulty with. I've seen people who are
> in similar jobs and they have very different titles: 'Senior health

promotion specialist for gay men', what does that mean? What would that say to people? . . . That sounds as if it's, you know, I'm up here, everyone else is down there. That I'm a professional first and foremost and only a gay man by chance. Um, I think when you over-professionalize this area of work you run into a problem where if you like you're denying grassroots activity, um, where you distance yourself from the grassroots. And in particular in this project, it's community development, we're supposed to be grassroots and bottom–up led, then, you know, calling yourself a professional constantly is not aiding that process at all.

K: Because its creating a sort of power difference or . . . ?

Yeah, and knowledge difference and everything really. You know, calling yourself a health professional to a lot of people is like, puts you on a level with a doctor, or it puts you well above what you are actually doing. Um, and I think that can only be negative.

Professionalism is really important to me, and I think more than anything my heart is with a kind of generation of, of gay male professionals who have expertise in sexual health . . . I want there to be a body of highly professionalized, actually, highly professionalized gay men with expertise in this field. I think there should be. That's what I want there to be. And that doesn't mean I don't believe in volunteerism or political activism . . . I'm really very taken by the notion of a whole body of knowledge and a whole body of expertise and a whole body of practice existing now where it didn't ten years ago. I find that very captivating somehow. And very inspiring. So I believe in professionalism more than anything.

Professionalism, Sex and Sexuality

In many ways the idea of being professional can be seen to exclude sex and sexuality. One example of this is that many people working in the field of sexuality have experienced difficulties in trying to get their work taken seriously (see Allgeier, 1984, and Fisher, 1989, for accounts of some of the difficulties sex researchers have faced), or have experienced ridicule and abuse. Similarly, those who have attempted to address issues relating to sexual boundaries within their professions have often found it impossible to conduct or report their research (see Brodsky, 1989; Rutter, 1991), or have faced hostility for daring to address the issue (Gechtman, 1989). Since sex has often been regarded as an illegitimate work topic, it is perhaps not surprising that issues about sex and sexuality have been difficult to validate as a professional concern. As the anthropologist Carol Vance writes (1991, p. 875):

> the discipline often appears to share the prevailing cultural view that sexuality is not an entirely legitimate area of study, and that such study necessarily casts doubt not only on the research but on the motives and character of the researcher . . . [there is a] clear message that sexuality is so dangerous an intellectual terrain it can ruin the careers of otherwise competent graduate students and academics.

As Brodsky (1989) notes, in some professions there has also long been an imperative not to have sex with clients.[2]

There is clearly, then, a sense in which the professional and the sexual are seen as excluding each other. This also applies to HIV-prevention outreach work. For example, even though the work involves discussing issues of sex and sexuality, working in sexualized environments, and being open about their own sexuality, many workers still found it hard to talk about boundary issues with managers for fear of being labelled unprofessional:

> I don't think I would feel able to go to the board of management and say: 'Look, I slept with someone who may be construed as a client', if I did. I just don't think I'd be able to do that. Whereas I think I should be able to. I think that would be a major knock really, I think, to how people would perceive my professionalism.

However, as is often the case, the view of sex, sexuality and professionalism as separate is problematic and contradictory, as professionalism and sex can also be seen to be intertwined. For example, the phrases being a 'professional' and the 'oldest profession' are both euphemisms for prostitution. Furthermore, tabloid newspapers continually sensationalize the sexual antics of professionals, and we all know what can happen on business trips! More recent sociological and psychological research has begun to highlight the links between sexuality and professionalism, for example in the growing literature on organizational sexuality and on sexual relationships between professionals and clients (Burrell, 1984; Hearn and Parkin, 1987; Hearn *et al.*, 1989; O'Gabbard, 1989).

Professionalism in the Context of Gay and Bisexual Men's HIV Prevention

In the case of HIV-prevention work with gay and bisexual men, there were particular twists which impacted on the more general relationship of professionalism, sex and sexuality. Such work takes place in a political and cultural climate that is generally not favourable to gay men. For workers there is always the possibility of a local scandal which could stop the work: this meant that many strongly felt the need to have what they did legitimized as work:

> ... because the work is very new and because of its highly sexual nature and because of its titillating sort of bits to it, unless we are seen, I think, as acting in the utmost professionalism then the work will be undervalued completely and people will see us as, you know, as a couple of gay boys having a good time on the poll tax or whatever.

By 'being professional', workers felt that they could gain acceptance for their work and would be taken seriously by other professionals. The fact that they were being paid to undertake the work was seen as of great importance in this respect.

Part of being professional was also seen to be about communicating the importance of the work. This involved demonstrating that outreach work was much more demanding than 'just hanging around with gay men in clubs', or 'being paid to go cruising'. As one worker said:

> That it's not just about going to a pub once a week, and you know spending six hours a week outside a cottage, it's about having things like boundaries, it's about time management, it's about administration, it's about having ideas, it's about following through those ideas, about having really shit meetings with people you can't stand ... it's about dealing with homophobia, it's about dealing with other professionals in the health service.

This reliance on an image of professionalism is a phenomenon which has also been highlighted by Cain (1994, p. 52) in a Canadian context:

> A professional image can help ... workers maintain a sense of competence and expertise in the face of the uncertainty surrounding the epidemic. It is hard to measure the success of their educational efforts, and in the absence of a cure for HIV, their support programs are often experienced as inadequate. By asserting that they are providers of a specialised and professional service, workers claim a status which is more highly valued than that afforded lay practitioners and peer counsellors. This image allows them to interact with doctors and social workers on a more equal footing and helps them successfully compete in an increasingly crowded field of AIDS service providers.

Being professional can be seen as a way to gain respect and support, as well as funds for the work. However, several workers felt ambiguous about being seen as professional. It is important to note that historically it has been 'the professions' that have criminalized and pathologized gay men. For example, it is not so long since the American Psychiatric Association categorized homo-sexuality as a mental disorder. It is perhaps therefore not surprising that many gay workers were also critical of professionalism and wary of describing themselves as professionals:

> To a certain extent as a gay man you teach yourself to mistrust authority. You teach yourself to mistrust certainly the NHS, and the police, and, um, your manager, and, uh, basically anybody straight . . . um, you basically learn to look after yourself. And to a certain extent there's this bloody great organization called X NHS Trust which is saying: 'No, you're not yourself, you are a very tiny cog in this very large organization and you will do as you are told' . . . I mean I am a gay man first and that's what I like to think and I really, I start to dig my heels in if anybody starts to try and undermine that.

In recent years this mistrust has at times been compounded by what has come to be described as the de-gaying of AIDS and the professionalization of the HIV field (Altman, 1986, 1994; Patton, 1990; King, 1993a, 1995) in which the involvement of professionals in the field, and links with the statu-tory sector, are seen to have had disastrous consequences for HIV-prevention work with gay men. The fact that for many gay men there is a clear link between both professionalism and discrimination (McNestry and Hartley, 1995, p. 8), as well as between professionalism and the neglect of gay men's needs, can create profound tensions for those workers who although having strong identities as gay men also view themselves as professional.

A further dimension to the relationship between professionalism and sexual identity is that most of the workers felt that because of the nature of the work their sexual and professional identities became fused.[3] For example, several of the workers described themselves as 'professional gay men':

> It's a sexual job and we're allowed to be a gay man. It's one of the few jobs where you're just allowed to be . . . I went to talk to, um, some probation officers and just sort of, you know, introduced my-self as a professional poof, and they looked very uncomfortable. They just didn't know whether I was like joking or not. I said: 'Well, yeah, I'm paid to be gay, I'm paid because of my experience of getting off with people in clubs . . . because without those skills, without having hung around clubs for years I wouldn't be able to do the work I'm doing now.'

This equation of the job with a certain sexual identity meant that some of the workers felt restrictions on telling those to whom they were not out as gay men, including relatives, their job titles. Several of the workers I spoke to were frustrated that being a professional and being a gay man were seen to be incompatible by others. This was the case both in terms of the perceptions of service users: 'And I think there's a bit of mistrust about like professional gay men because it's somehow like, within the political gay community it's like "Oh, they've sold themselves short to social services", or whatever' and other professionals who, for example, would suggest that gay men are all obsessed with having sex. Being seen as inherently sexual, the workers felt that their gay identity often overrode their identity as a professional. Not because they wished it to be this way, but because this was how they were viewed by other professionals. Therefore, they felt there was extra pressure put on them to be professional and maintain sexual boundaries. As one worker said:

> I was on an interview panel and one of the questions was 'How do you think the notion of boundaries relates to a gay men's HIV-prevention officer?' . . . I should have challenged [it], I wanted to say 'No, it should be how does it relate to health promotion, an HIV-prevention officer?' . . . sometimes I feel there's a subtext that gay men are just very promiscuous basically and need reigning in. Whether it's true or not it is a bit offensive in a way because . . . if there was pressure for me to have a code of conduct for my post I would say 'No, I have professional conduct and unless the whole department is bound by that I don't see [why] my work [should be].'

This sexualization of gay men has also been pointed out by Parkin and Green (1994) in their work on sexuality in residential-care settings. Here, they found that gay male care workers' sexuality was frequently seen to be 'problematic, predatory and paedophile', and gay male workers kept their sexuality hidden or put up with homophobia and sexual innuendo from colleagues. This prejudice from colleagues was also mentioned by some of the men I spoke to:

> We've often had discussions [in the department] where I've suddenly felt actually my whole identity and way of life is being discussed, like one member of staff said to me: 'Oh, you know, I actually have a lot of negative feelings around homosexuals.'

For this reason several of the workers felt that they were under pressure to represent the gay community in a good light to other professionals.

Finally, gay workers also felt they were subject to criticism for being too personally involved in their work. The fact that one of the women I interviewed felt that their service was seen as being more professional because women were involved, rather than just affected gay men, highlights the difficulties gay men may have in being accepted as professional. As Altman (1993) points out, gay men who play a role as community representatives run the risk of both distancing themselves from the gay community and being seen by others to be biased if they speak out (Griffiths, 1995).

Professionalism as Cultural Construct

One of the striking features of the interview data was the emphasis many workers placed on the phrase 'being professional'. When questioned about what this meant, workers came up with different answers, though some common themes were identifiable. Many found it hard to give a specific definition which seems to parallel the loose way that the term is used. As one worker said:

> What does being professional mean? Well, I don't know. It's just really difficult, isn't it? Some professions have a guide of ethics, have a code of conduct, so it might mean adhering to that, but I'm not involved in a profession like a lawyer, or a doctor, or a teacher, or a counsellor . . . But being professional is used in a blanket way, and it's used to mean anything, from meaning you get your mail out really efficiently and quickly, you know: 'Very professional', to meaning what we're talking about sexual boundaries.

It is interesting in this quote that the distinction between 'the professions' and the more cultural idea of 'being professional' is highlighted. Much of the existing sociological work on professions and professionalism takes a macro- or structural approach (Macdonald, 1995). Here, the focus is on how groups of people professionalize, or how professions can be defined: which occupations count as true professions. In contrast the theme that has emerged from this research centres on professionalism as cultural practice, that is, on how people use the term professional, and what images being professional conjures up at the level of everyday discourse.

Although undertaking this research has probably sensitized me to the frequent use of the terms 'professional', 'unprofessional' and 'professionalism', it is clearly a construct that is drawn on in a wide range of contexts and used frequently in everyday language. For example, the following are a few references which I have noted recently:

> Marilyn was now freebasing cocaine regularly, which might have explained his deficient logic. He swore blind that he wasn't basing before he went on stage at Area [a New York club]: 'I would never do that, it's unprofessional.' (Boy George/Bright, 1995, p. 271)

> PROFESSIONAL, ATTRACTIVE, slim male, honest and genuine. Seeks similar female for walks, talks, pubs and lunch. Letter, photo. Box 524. (*Time Out*, 1995, Talking Hearts, p. 159)

> [Dr] Margoulies punctuated the thought with an innocent tweak of Bull's clitoris . . . From here on in everything that the good doctor

did was tantamount to taking a chainsaw to his Tree of Knowledge. For Margoulies had abandoned his professional perspectives, he had allowed his own likes and dislikes to affect his judgement. He was no longer acting in the best interests of his patient. (Self, 1993, p. 127)

It is interesting to note from these examples that the word 'professional' is used to refer both to identity and a set of behaviours or practices. So, for example, in the quotes above we can see it being referred to as rules or ideas about how professionals should behave: not taking drugs, not having sexual contact with patients, not acting in your own interest, and as an identity marker, signalling characteristics such as respectability, wealth, career, and being too busy working to find sexual partners. This distinction is important because it illuminates the way in which being professional not only says something about what people do but also about who they are. In this regard it is interesting to reflect on the parallels with sexual identity (Weeks, 1995).

Many of those interviewed found defining 'professional' quite difficult. People frequently said that it was something they had never really thought about before, even though they recognized that they often used the term. Table 10.1 identifies some of the issues mentioned in relation to being professional. It is interesting to compare these definitions with the key characteristics that Williams (1993, p. 8) notes are often cited by those attempting to identify key traits that characterize professions:

- skill based on theoretical knowledge;
- the provision of training and occupation;
- tests of the competence of members;
- organization;
- adherence to a professional code of conduct; and
- altruistic service.

Clearly these two lists are very different. Indeed, comparing the two it would seem that possibly only the last two items on William's list would be seen to be relevant to the items mentioned by interviewees and listed in Table 10.1. For example, in the table no attention is paid to things such as specialized knowledge which sociologically are usually seen as defining professions. Instead there is a focus on the mechanics of actually carrying out the work and reference to the organizational settings in which work takes place. Significantly the list also addresses the emotional work (Hochschild, 1983; Star, 1989) involved in being a professional.

For the workers interviewed, being professional seemed to be defined mainly in relation to behavioural characteristics and the way in which work is carried out. In this respect the image of professionals was something that was frequently mentioned. For example, one worker's response to the question 'What does being a professional mean?' was: 'Mm, being professional. Being paid a good salary and having a smart title!' A significant amount of

Table 10.1 *Definitions of the term professional*

Definitions generated from interviews	Examples given in interviews
Focusing on a task	Having a clear plan about what you are doing, why and with whom; clear aim; knowing what the work involves and what you need to do; setting objectives.
Providing a service	Providing a service well
Equitable service delivery	Being non-judgmental; contacting a wide variety of people
Boundaries	Not displaying inappropriate behaviour e.g. drinking alcohol; adherence to a code of conduct; not having sex with clients; not expecting needs for sex and intimacy to be met through work; a private life that doesn't denigrate work; clear boundaries; not having sex; confidentiality
Living the job	Identity/vocation
Being responsible	Being responsible to communities/users; responsible to funders; explaining your actions to people; instilling confidence in others
Being credible to a wide range of people	Looking smart
Ensuring that resources are used effectively	Using resources well
Tailoring work	Adapting to different people/ environments; using correct language; dressing appropriately
Detachment	Controlling feelings; being appropriately emotional; not reacting personally; not bringing personal issues into the work; not being rude to people; not hugging or kissing people as a greeting at work; not losing temper; keeping distance and not being one of the lads; maintaining neutrality; avoid 'bitchy' comments when socializing
Being paid	
Aware of relationship to wider system	Line management and forms; public role; using supervision and action plans

Table 10.1 *(cont.)*

Definitions generated from interviews	Examples given in interviews
Access to privileged information	
Having knowledge which you have to impart	Power to use information; using information to help others
Doing the best you can	Giving best advice; confident in your information; learning when to say no/ your limits; eliciting information without upsetting people; getting mail out quickly; finding out information you don't know; being aware of how you are working
Authoritative role	Authority; being competent; having a smart title; theory behind work; upholding what the project stands for
Being ethical	Respecting confidentiality
Responding to needs	
Promote needs of communities by working with and empowering them	

people also mentioned the importance of appropriate dress, something also noted by Cain (1994).

The fact that these lists are different helps highlight some of the tensions workers experienced between traditional notions of what being professional meant and how they wanted to work, or what they valued. In order to explore some of these differences in more detail, the remainder of this chapter is divided into sections addressing some of the different definitions of being professional already outlined. Through a closer examination of these I illuminate some of the reasons why professionalism and sexual identity sometimes have a problematic relationship in HIV-related work.

'Walk It Like You Talk It' – Experience, Expertise and Knowledge

Professions have been defined as knowledge-based occupations (Larson, 1977). Although sociologically, health services are often described as semi-professions, and thus not seen as true professions, it still seems useful to reflect on the idea of HIV-prevention as a knowledge-based occupation. This may be revealing about the term professional and the apparent contradictions it causes in the HIV field.

One of the immediate questions raised through the interviews was the difference between taught knowledge and life experience. The former is classically seen to be a defining feature of professionals and the latter was frequently mentioned as the primary qualification for those doing HIV-prevention work with gay men. Is there a difference between knowledge and experience? One way to stimulate thought about this is to look at existing definitions and current uses of words. The *Collins English Dictionary* (1990) defines the primary current meaning of experienced as 'having become skilful or knowledgeable from extensive contact or participation or observation', and defines experience as meaning 'direct personal participation or observation; actual knowledge or contact . . . accumulated knowledge, experience of practical matters'. This latter definition is interesting because it is suggestive both of a link between experience and knowledge, and the variety of ways in which knowledge can be gained through experience. It emphasizes contact and participation, the major qualifications which many men suggested they brought to the work through their life experience as gay or bisexual men. However, while knowledge through contact, participation and observation was also brought to the work by women, for example, by being part of the lesbian and gay community, by having gay friends or through direct learning from gay men, women rarely emphasized their experience in the same way.

Consider next a current dictionary definition of knowledge:

> knowledge – the facts, feelings or experiences known by a person or a group of people . . . awareness, consciousness or familiarity gained by experience or learning . . . informed learning, specific information about a subject. (Collins English Dictionary, 1990)

This identifies learning, something which refers back to a key trait that has been used to characterize professions: training and skill based on theoretical knowledge. It is the possession of an expert, systematized and theoretical body of knowledge which is seen as vital for any occupation wishing to professionalize. As Macdonald (1995, pp. 2–3) writes:

> The lay person has no means of knowing objectively whether the professional can in fact provide the service on offer, and must therefore make a judgement on other criteria. In fact the professional has to be taken on trust and so is keen to display those characteristics which are believed to represent trustworthiness. These will include evidence of training and knowledge acquired – degrees, diplomas and certificates.

Because of the historical (and in some cases continued) discrimination by professions, such characteristics are not necessarily going to be seen as signs of trust by gay and bisexual men (King, 1995). Indeed, it is more likely that trust will be signalled through shared identity or sexual practice, as well as through symbols that signify a link to sex with men and/or the gay community. Indeed, it is partly because of an historically poor or non-existent relationship with the lesbian and gay community, that in Britain at least the statutory sector has needed to work with voluntary and gay community organizations in order to undertake effective HIV-prevention. In terms of the recent rise in gay and bisexual men's work, there are positive examples of statutory organizations appointing gay men because they recognize the need for workers to have a good understanding of the diversity of gay and bisexual culture. In this sense there is a positive endorsement of the vital skills and knowledge gay men can bring to an organization. On the more negative side, such appointments may enable organizations to continue to ignore the need to work with gay men, by seeing this solely as the province of the gay men's worker. This can lead to individual workers being very isolated and gaining little organizational support.

It is not surprising that workers themselves saw sexual identity as crucially important. As one worker said: being gay is 'our expertise'. Many of the men talked about being employed because they *were* gay men, rather than in relation to other skills they may have, and several cited their sexual identity as the most important job qualification:

> I suppose one of the qualifications that I have for this job is the fact that I'm a young gay man, you know, and that's something that was important to the project when they appointed me, um, you know . . . My life experience is qualification in itself, and, you know, and my anger, and my emotional response are qualifications. You know what I mean? And so it's about, you know, it's actually recognizing human elements, rather than just sort of like working within a framework of like, you know sort of like, you know academia.

> If it wasn't for my sexual identity I wouldn't be doing the work.

This is quite different from the usual idea of expertise gained through professional training and formal qualifications. In this occupation what qualified you to do the job was life experience and insights gained from a gay sexual identity. This situation was seen to be positive because it recognized the importance of community-based work and the need for culturally appropriate and rooted HIV-prevention initiatives.

It is interesting that it is particular life experience that is seen to qualify one to undertake sexual health promotion with gay men, rather than health-promotion expertise. It would be useful to discover how this relates to other areas of health promotion or care. Equally, the question could be asked: why do many of those with health-promotion expertise not necessarily feel qualified to work with gay men? Unfortunately, there is no space to address these issues here.

Several of the men I interviewed felt that sexuality as a qualification generated difficulties. For example, emphasizing the link between life experience and identity resulted in knowledge becoming essentialized as an automatic consequence of sexual identity. As not all gay men have had the same life experiences, some workers felt that such appeals to authenticity and shared experience led to a neglect of the variety and diversity of gay and bisexual men's experiences (Altman, 1993, p. 5; Deverell and Prout, 1995; Prout and Deverell, 1995; Sandfort, 1995). For example, some suggested that the re-gaying of AIDS had in fact led to the 'Sohoization'[4] of the epidemic where certain gay men's needs and desires had become reified as *all* gay men's. The re-gaying of AIDS was also seen to have led to reductionist arguments about who is actually qualified to do the work. This has resulted in women, who have historically been involved in HIV-prevention with gay and bisexual men, feeling that they are no longer seen to have valid skills and knowledge to offer because their genitals do not fit (Williams, 1994).

The idea of an automatic link between knowledge and identity was also seen to mask the fact that gay men had also gone through a process of learning. As one woman worker described, reflecting on her experience at having been taught how to cruise by two gay male friends:

> I mean they pick it up, just like I picked it up. You know, you either go on site with somebody who's done it before and you learn, or you go on site and you observe . . . I mean, it's not inbred in people you know, it's observed, it's learned.

Indeed, a few of the men I interviewed described how they had had to learn to cruise themselves. Some talked about how, before their employment, they had not had personal experience of certain activities such as anal sex or public sex environments, even though they were assumed to have had them.

Although most people interviewed felt that having a gay or bisexual identity, or at least having sex with men, was an important experience to bring to the job, many pointed out that there was a need to emphasize the other qualities needed for outreach work, and for those doing this work to feel validated in the other skills they had. As many workers emphasized, not all gay men make good outreach workers, and there is a need to understand that knowledge and expertise can be gained in different ways.

Both a Client and a Professional – Non-distanced Relationships

Despite an interest in appearing professional, the construct of professionalism was something that was questioned by many workers, for as gay men they were themselves part of the client group and many had an emotional and political motivation for doing the job:

> the reason why I got into this job was because I had a keen interest in seeing HIV-prevention done among gay men, because I'd seen what had been happening and it had all been really negative, and because politically I wanted to be involved in a job that had something to say to me personally, something that gave me some kind of personal fulfilment, and about which I knew a lot, because I've been involved in like, gay politics and gay organizations for a long time.

For many, the primary reason for becoming involved was to work with gay men, and their feelings of empathy with clients and service users meant that sometimes they did not feel a great distinction between themselves and those with whom they worked:

> Um, I think the nature of the work concerned it's like, because you're working with men who have sex with men and you are yourself a man who has sex with men and so on, a lot of the issues . . . are issues that concern you as well not just because you're working . . . because a lot of the people who [you] come into contact with are like yourself, and there's a kind of obligation . . . particularly as a Black worker working in a Black project for men who have sex with men, it's like this, you know minority within a minority, really. Um, you do feel this duty really to do the work . . . it's almost like if you weren't being paid you'd feel this duty to do it, because it's about helping your own people, you know.

At times the worker's identity as a professional was therefore less strong than other identities related, for example, to their sexuality or ethnicity. This meant that their relationships with service users were very different from those considered to be the norm for other professionals. As Williams (1993, p. 8) writes:

> An important element of the professional-client relationship, it is proposed, is that of 'mystification': professionals promote their services as esoteric. They create dependence on their skills and reduce the areas of knowledge and experience they have in common with their clients. In this way they increase the 'social distance' between themselves and their clients, and so gain increasing autonomy.

The workers were not interested in increasing distance between themselves and service users/clients but in working on the basis of a shared sexual identity – or at least the shared experience of having sex with men. As part of the client group the workers were in fact potential consumers as well as providers of services, an issue rarely considered in studies of professionalism. Whether or not as part of the client group workers do have a thorough understanding of gay and bisexual men's needs is an interesting question. This could usefully be the subject of further research, particularly given the recent policy emphasis on the role of consumers in healthcare.

There is an obvious difference in the workers' roles to many other professionals. The workers I interviewed are not paid by clients for a service, and go out offering services to people, rather than being approached. This meant that their relationships often took on a different dynamic. As one worker said:

> I think when you are doing outreach on the scene and things like that people are really, mm, they see you as one of them. If you are doing it in an office, if somebody comes to you in an office, you are a professional worker, do you know what I mean? It's that difference. And the power structure seems different, the power relationship feels different, it seems you're on a more of an equal level if you are out in a club.

Indeed, given the nature of the places they worked in, several workers suggested that different definitions of what it meant to be professional needed to be adopted. For example, you could still be professional while being naked, wearing jeans, or drinking beer in a bar.

The Personal is Professional

A further issue identified in relation to professionalism concerned not bringing personal issues into the work. This form of behaviour is frequently associated with the idea of being professional. For example, in the novel *The Remains of the Day*, the butler character, Stevens, discusses what distinguishes a great butler from a merely competent butler. It is, he argues, a matter of dignity:

> 'dignity' has to do crucially with a butler's ability not to abandon the professional being he inhabits. Lesser butlers will abandon their professional being for the private one at the least provocation. For such persons, being a butler is like playing some pantomime role; a small push, a slight stumble, and the façade will drop off to reveal the actor underneath. The great butlers are great by virtue of their ability to inhabit their professional role and inhabit it to the utmost; they will not be shaken out by external events, however surprising, alarming or vexing. (Ishiguro, 1990, pp. 42–3)

This idea of professionalism was clearly internalized by some of the workers, who strove to keep their personal views and feelings out of work. This involved such things as trying to remain non-judgmental and provide an equitable service to all those worked with, even when they did not like them or they made offensive comments; not shouting in meetings; concentrating on the needs of those worked with; and not displaying sexual excitement. In this respect, several workers talked about the need to distinguish their role as workers:

> My line is that if I'm working on the streets in a sense my sexuality is secondary to being a worker, and though I use my sexuality I'm there as a worker, not necessarily as a gay man . . . I know that with that pay packet and with that contract comes a responsibility and that responsibility includes not having sex with those people [I work with].

However, there was also a feeling that to do community-based work there was a need to draw on personal experience and motivation:

> I'm not just standing there spouting about what the textbook says, um, I'm a real person, with real feelings and a real sex life. Um, and I think there can be too much detachment which is why I'm always testing things out . . . things like lubricants, I'll always be able to recommend to people which ones I think are the best.

> this work relies on being more than professional . . . it's got to do with what I was saying about vocation, and I think you've got to do it with vigour and with enthusiasm and, uh, with passion . . . I suppose I see being professional as being a basic set of core, like ethical, being ethical if you like, um, but I don't think this work will succeed if you're just that.

Many workers emphasized the importance of having community links and were concerned that a professional image might distance them from the men with whom they worked. For many of the gay workers, being part of the local community and being seen to have had similar experiences and difficulties was the way in which they built trust. This led some to suggest that there was a need for a new definition of professionalism, one which recognized the usefulness of shared experience:

> it's about other people appreciating where, where the normal, or what's conceived to be the accepted boundaries, are sometimes not always the accepted boundaries between gay workers and gay clients . . . It's where the clients will need you to relate to them in a framework other than the straight world, or where, for example, the subtext of where you both socialize comes in, or the slang words you might both use, do you know what I mean? Or the kind of similar oppression that you're both subjected to, similar discriminations that you've both had, where you're just going to have to acknowledge that within the counselling relationship, or within the professional relationship,

and it does change, it has a different texture to it . . . the boundaries need to be kept in check really tightly, but I think gay workers, that I've seen, good gay workers have been able to judge when and where to relax them just so far without confusing the clients, to use that to their benefit.

Although at times very valuable, being close to those worked with could prove difficult. In this respect, the workers' experiences were similar to others doing community development work in small or bounded communities (Cruikshank, 1989). However, at times the workers' stresses were much more specific, particularly when working with men who were experiencing similar anxieties. For example:

I used to think that I could work with HIV issues quite, in a detached sense, in a really relevant way, that I could relate to issues. It was like so far away from me that, I'd be able to work in a really professional way with it. I've kind of got a lot more involved with my own personal issues . . . really worried about my own [HIV] status and testing issues and all that kind of thing. And, um, maybe now I feel that I'm at my most ineffective in relation to HIV work.

Interestingly, there is a move in many of the semi-professions (health promotion, social work and nursing) towards a new understanding of professionalism. This has involved the challenging of expert knowledge and a recognition of the importance of the 'self' or personal qualities of the professional, most particularly in their interpersonal skills and intuition (Williams, 1993). The development of a new understanding in which the personal is seen to be a potential resource for professionals may make the adoption of a professional identity sit more comfortably for many. However, it still raises issues about how much the personal experiences, values and feelings of the worker should influence what is done.

One of Us, One of Them, or One of Those – Payment and Professionalization

Interestingly, one of the most commonly understood meanings of professionalism does not appear in Williams' list, although it does in the list generated by those I spoke to: that is the equation of being professional with being paid. The fact that at the level of cultural understanding, being professional means being paid is illuminating of a major tension for many gay men in HIV work. As their primary motivation for doing the work is linked to a political and altruistic desire to prevent more gay men from becoming infected, rather than developing a career or being paid, labelling themselves as professional symbolizes something directly at odds with this motivation. Although most of those I interviewed enjoyed having a salary, most would actively resist seeing payment as their reason for being in the field. This unease is clearly related to wider debates within HIV work about professionalism and the professionalization of AIDS voluntary organizations. For example, there has long been a cynicism about people who are merely 'AIDS professionals' rather than personally committed to the work. Sometimes this has extended to a distrust of heterosexuals or even those who are HIV-negative (Kennett, 1995) as the following comments underline:

> I mean I had some really bad experiences when I first got involved in this work, with like certain people that were working within different agencies, and I was made to feel very, very guilty . . . not so much guilty about being negative, but more about, 'Well, you don't know how lucky you are,' and, you know, 'What can you possibly know, you can't possibly know what it's like to live with this virus. To have to make decisions based on this virus,' and, you know, 'You're coming in here and you know you want to get things done well, you don't know,' you know what I mean? And that was very hard to work that one through, because it's about . . . it's like, you know, legitimizing your existence.

> that's when I think being a woman, a straight woman, means that you're somehow up for it as well, to be attacked in some ways . . . one thing I've had said is, you know, 'Who do you think you are, heterosexual woman running a service about HIV when it's gay men that are dying, what do you know?', that kind of stuff . . . so, you know, in a way you are a target for that because you, because you can't use that thing: 'Well, it's my community, too, you know, I'm a gay man so I'm an infected or affected person too.' Um, you know you sort of lose that option.

This emphasis on personal experience can also be seen in the way that credibility in the HIV field sometimes appears to stem from relating the number of people that you have known to have died from HIV disease. Furthermore, the assumed link between sexual identity and personal experience of HIV means that assumptions are made about who has been personally affected and who has not:

> Straight people and women have their grief around HIV as well, but, um, but, um, that's not assumed about you, I think . . . There's more often the assumption that you're doing it because it's a good job, or you're CV collecting or whatever, rather than personal commitment you know. I think there's a lot of that.

In part, this situation may have developed from the roots of HIV-prevention being in volunteerism and activism, and within the West specifically having emerged from within the lesbian and gay community (Altman, 1986; Patton, 1990). In this sense, then, 'professional' highlights the distinction between those who are paid to do the work and volunteers.

There is an understandable anger that at the beginning of the epidemic the only prevention and education that took place was through gay community organizing – and yet when professionals became involved they often took credit for what had been done. This background has led to a situation in which the term 'professional' is often used to refer not just to those who are paid, but to those who are not truly committed to the cause and just interested in their careers. Several people mentioned that within the HIV field a common way to disparage someone's work or question their commitment has been to label them 'too professional'. As one interviewee commented, 'Professional is a hurtful word.' It is therefore not surprising that some people do not feel happy embracing it:

> I can think of so many projects ... where [gay] workers have not been committed to anything but their own careers, and that the service, and, you know, the development of services has been ignored ... that to me, you know, is the professional gay men syndrome which is why I'm so defensive when I'm labelled as that.

Some of these issues have come to the fore in arguments about the re-gaying of AIDS. For example in an article describing sexual boundaries as unnecessarily professional and bureaucratic, King (1993b, p. 14) argues that boundaries are a manifestation of the de-gaying and professionalization of AIDS organizations, where gay identity has become secondary to professional identity:

> In the mid-1980s, when safer sex campaigns led to unprecedented behaviour changes among gay men, understanding and spreading the word about safer sex was something that any gay man could do in his everyday life. But in the de-gaying years, AIDS education came to be seen as a job for professional employees. In the unusual event of any HIV-prevention campaigns being targeted at gay men, safer sex education became something done to gay men by nine-to-five experts working to codes of conduct.

This criticism has also been taken up by British organizations such as Gay Men Fighting AIDS (GMFA), an organization set up to do prevention work specifically for gay men. The following is an extract from an early newsletter:

> GMFA has caused a bit of a stir with our very personal way of promoting safer sex. Unlike some other organizations, we don't forbid our volunteers from having sex with 'clients'. Indeed, we see it as

the essential way gay men can promote safer sex. We don't see ourselves as separate from other gay men, rather we see ourselves as part of a community and as part of a safer sex movement within that community.

This seems to have rattled some outsiders who are confused by our 'professional boundaries'. The implication is that our priorities and responsibilities are unclear. While they may be unclear to people outside GMFA, they seem clear enough to our volunteers. We agree to put the project first . . . we don't spend the whole time in bushes demonstrating blow jobs. We save that for tea breaks. (Dockrell, 1993)

This emphasis on being part of the community has upset some other gay men's workers who also feel very much part of the community but do not have the same freedom as GMFA. For example, as health authority employees, many are subject to codes of conduct. All the workers I interviewed were also very concerned not to do anything that might bring their project into disrepute and thus affect the continuity of the work. This was particularly the case because having fought hard for funding for gay men's work they did not want to endanger the work through having sex with men who could be construed as clients. As one worker said in response to GMFA's criticism:

I mean they've set up this thing about, you know, the normal boring HIV professionals who don't agree with that model and we who know. When actually the normal boring HIV-prevention workers know that they want people to tell their lovers and, of course, want people to have sex, but what they know is that for paid workers in that formal set-up to do that . . . is not necessarily ethical and is generally not practical.

These articles were mentioned by several of those I interviewed who felt unfairly criticized, and upset that their identity as gay men was being overlooked because they were paid and worked in the statutory sector. As paid workers they did not have the same freedoms as GMFA volunteers, but they wanted their experience and commitment as gay men to be recognized. Many were frustrated at the division between professionals and gay men because they felt they were both. One worker suggested that a way forward was to distinguish between the different roles of volunteers, activists and professionals:

I guess what I'm saying is somehow, it's something like, well, let's just accept that we're professionals. We are professionals in the sense that we're paid to do this job, and we're paid to do it to certain standards, and somehow I think it's disingenuous to pretend that we're not. Now then, I think the question facing volunteers and political activists is different.

This situation outlines some of the tensions that have developed within a field that historically has grown out of the work of volunteers and those affected by the epidemic, and has increased and changed dramatically in terms of management, bureaucracy and paid posts (Weeks, Taylor-Laybourn and Aggleton, 1994). As the majority of people working in the HIV-prevention field are now paid, the distinction between commitment and career seems inadequate. However, the strength of feeling that the word 'professional' can arouse highlights the need to recognize the major role that personal commitment, community involvement and politics still play in the work.

'It's the Condom Man' – The Merging of Professional and Sexual Identity

One final issue to emerge from considering the relationship between sexual identity and professionalism is the vocational aspect of the work, the identity element of being professional which I suggested earlier. In the last few years, with the increase in work targeted at gay and bisexual men, there has been a corresponding rise in gay and bisexual men's workers. This has led some to suggest that the HIV-prevention worker has become a new figure on the gay scene: as visible and identifiable perhaps as leather queens, drag queens or clones. As Harrison (1995, p. 55) describes it:

> I can usually spot one a mile off. It's something to do with his haircut, the style of his clothes, and the ubiquitous shoulder bag which seems to accompany him everywhere.

Several of the workers I interviewed also joked about the developing image of the HIV outreach worker. Furthermore, workers talked a lot about becoming identified locally through their work and how their identification as a worker marked them out from the rest of the gay community. This was particularly the case for those working in smaller towns. As one worker put it: 'You're always known for your work rather than, say, for example, the size of your dick (laughs), which is what most other men on the scene are known about.'

Therefore when socializing, many of the men reported that they were always seen as a worker rather than just another gay man. This identification of the workers by others often went further, with people making assumptions about their HIV status. For example:

> I get the feeling that a certain amount of what we do sort of inhibits people from talking to us ... I mean, it's always been a bit of a laughing joke really, in the fact that we're theoretically some of the

most connected and well-known gay men in the whole of, in the whole city and yet in reality we're always the people stood on our own in the club! . . . I mean, in terms of your social life, you're always tainted with the fact that you're an AIDS worker . . . so it's not always like the great advantage, you know, in terms of meeting sexual partners.

If you work for an HIV agency people always think you have HIV . . . and it does fucking ruin your sex life because they won't approach you because they think you're HIV-positive.

This meant that workers would often not be approached when socializing on their local gay scene outside work. It was also sometimes hard to encourage contact during work sessions as men would fear identifying themselves as HIV-positive, or as having a concern if their friends saw them talking to a worker. This raises interesting issues for community-based ways of working.

Not surprisingly, everyone I interviewed felt that doing the work had had an impact on their own sex lives. Specifically, several people talked about the fact that their professional identity often carried through to their own sex lives:

It's like they're putting a condom on and they were going: 'God, I was convinced you were going to look at me when I was doing that!' You know. And I'm going, well, you know: 'No I wasn't looking and I'm not interested,' you know, whatever. I mean that really brings it home to you. You've got to the stage here, you're in a very intimate situation with one person and they're like having kittens because you might be looking at how they're putting a condom on . . . If you've got to that stage, you'd think that they'd have put your occupation to one side, but it's not always the case.

I very rarely sleep with men in this city and that is for all sorts of reasons . . . a lot of it is about fear that they want to have sex with me because of my job. You know 'Mr Safer Sex' and all that stuff, and the other fear is that they may tell other people in the city what I'm like in bed, really, and this is this person who keeps saying how wonderful safer sex is and how erotic it is and they may not find me very erotic at all, find me quite a bore! That feels, you know, that feels quite difficult.

Well I think that this work has had quite a profound effect in my sexual relationships, and I mean, I mean I don't know but I've some-times had the feeling that people who sleep with me are reminded of their own mortality and of AIDS, because that's the work that I do . . . I mean that has happened mid-sex you know, all of a sudden there's a bit of anxiety and it's like, am I their partner or am I their counsellor?

In larger towns, the situation was slightly different. Here, workers described how they had started to socialize mainly with other gay men involved in HIV-prevention. This led some to suggest that they had become separated from the experiences and needs of other gay men:

> You become part of a community of workers, and a kind of culture of HIV work, and become kind of socialized into that. Where it's very easy to talk about sex, comparatively very easy to be gay, very. Well, maybe not easy to have an HIV test, that's ridiculous, but it's part of your social currency that people may have HIV tests, you know, and have comparatively good support around, around sexual health. And that's a boundary that also needs addressing. Now it's very easy to sit and sort of wave the flag of authenticity and say 'Well, what about the real gay men out there?' and all that stuff, but I do think that needs paying some attention to really.

This was a situation where over-reliance on personal experience was thought to be potentially very damaging in terms of providing appropriate services. This was particularly the case because, as some suggested, many other gay and bisexual men do not prioritize HIV-prevention as their major need, and in fact may have other more pressing needs which they would like addressed. Because of their focus on HIV, workers may overestimate its perceived importance among other gay men.

Many of the workers felt that they were 'living the job' and talked about their personal and professional lives being very linked. For example:

> I'm conscious that my actions are limited. In some ways I mean, if I go and act like a complete prat at a club, it's going to be difficult to go back and enter that environment again as a professional ... for that reason you never stop working.

> It's stressful because you are ... the interface between the gay community and the social services and health authority, education [department] whatever, so you're constantly responsible for your actions whenever you're in professional arenas. And you're also aware of the fact that you're working in a project when you're out in the gay scene as well, do you know what I mean? You still carry that responsibility with you all the time. You know there isn't a big distinction between the personal and the professional.

Again, this was much more of an issue in smaller towns where workers had to work and socialize in the same places. Indeed, where there was a small and closely networked scene, the workers felt that their own sexual experiences had the potential to damage their professional identity. For example, several workers mentioned feeling a great pressure to always have safer sex. This was an area where they felt it was impossible to draw a personal and professional boundary; if it became known that they had unsafe sex, their professionalism would be seriously challenged.

What these crossovers highlight are the identity aspects of being a professional. Being a professional was not just seen to be about behaving in particular ways at particular times but to some extent was about having a permanent work-related identity:

> You're a gay man in your social life, you're also a gay man professionally . . . and there never seems to be this let off of something completely different from what you do . . . you never really leave your job at work in some respects. You know, you feel as if your life is being paid for by the health authority.

Some workers suggested that becoming 'the condom man' was comparable to other professionals, such as doctors, who in some senses are never off-duty. As gay men's workers it was felt that such crossovers were even more striking as their sexual and professional identities were clearly linked:

> when some people label you a professional gay man . . . when you hear comments like that you just find them really irritating that, that people can't see that . . . your work's about more than just you being gay and you bring other skills and attributes, or what have you. And yet, you know, at the end of the day you know that you're there because you're a gay man. It's very confusing.

Because of the nature of the work and the importance attached to their own sexual identities, for gay men their sexual and professional identities were complexly intertwined.

Conclusions

This chapter has explored some of the issues that have arisen for gay men's workers in relation to 'being professional'. Although not seeing themselves as a profession, the workers clearly drew on cultural notions of what being professional meant and emphasized the importance of being seen to be professional. To some extent this was linked to the new health service culture in Britain and the need to be seen to be professional in order to successfully compete for services. Being professional was also seen as a good defence against attacks from the tabloid press or others.

However, many workers felt ambivalent about labelling themselves professional and some actively resisted it. This was because of such things as the historical development of HIV-prevention; the discrimination against gay men by professions; the importance of community-based ways of working; and a desire not to be detached and distanced. The contradictions and anxieties this produced made it very difficult for those workers who, although having strong identities as gay men, also viewed themselves as professionals. Having to retain credibility both among other professionals and other gay and bisexual men, while still maintaining their own sense of integrity and political commitment, could be very stressful.

Developing roles in a new occupational field, the workers were to some extent caught up in a process of defining appropriate professional conduct. Trying to do this in a field that has consistently challenged professional groups and notions of professionalism proved hard. This was particularly the case given that the term 'professional' has been used very disparagingly in HIV work, and been used to criticize people for a multitude of 'sins', such as being heterosexual, being paid, having qualifications or working for the statutory sector. Although these factors may be related, and at times overlap, they are significantly different. Arguably too many issues have been hidden under the term 'professional'. It is therefore unfortunate that important arguments about the neglect of gay men's needs and the need for community-based work with gay and bisexual men have at times been confused with a rejection of anything that is seen to be related to being professional.

As the connotations of being professional identified in the course of the study show, aspects of being professional were seen to be important to developing new services and carrying out work successfully. Indeed, some interviewees saw being professional as a way to improve services for gay and bisexual men and to get the needs of gay and bisexual men recognized more widely. Given that many workers spoke about the different responsibilities placed on them as paid workers, further exploration of what it might mean to be a professional HIV worker may be useful. This may in turn create further understanding of the role of paid workers in community-based work, and provide support for those who walk the fine line between 'selling themselves short' and being 'too personally involved'.

The development within the health services of a new model for professional practice, away from expert and theoretical knowledge to support interpersonal skills, provides scope for the development of a more useful notion of professionalism. This could embrace such things as the importance of knowledge gained through personal experience, workers' political commitment and community involvement.

Whatever the case, given the frequency with which the term 'professional' is used, and the fact that it is a highly loaded term that carries many diverse meanings, more reflection on its perceived relationship to work and sexual identity would be useful. This is particularly important considering that different understandings of what it means to be professional continue to guide HIV-prevention practice.

Acknowledgments

I am grateful to The HIV Project, London, for giving me the time to write this paper, and to Chris Bonell, Jason Annetts and Mark Bitel for useful comments and support.

Notes

1 The study involved 25 in-depth semi-structured interviews carried out between 1992 and 1995. Interviews took place with HIV-prevention workers in various towns and cities throughout England. The research also involved participant observation, group discussion and documentary analysis.
2 It is only relatively recently that this has been codified or legislated against. Indeed, although there is often an unspoken rule that sex with clients is unethical or unprofessional, not all professional codes explicitly address this issue. Indeed, Rutter (1991) in his study of sexual encounters between therapists and clients has argued that such professional codes do not deter sex taking place, and may even psychologically encourage it by presenting it as forbidden.
3 Although this may seem unusual, using one's sexuality is often an expected but unspoken part of the job for many women. Adkins (1992), Pringle (1988) and others have shown how women are often employed for their sexuality and are expected to use it. One of the differences is that women's sexuality is assumed, and expected, to be heterosexual even when it may not be. Women's sexuality is also rarely an openly cited and coded job qualification.
4 Soho is an area of London that has become popular among certain lesbians and gay men. During the late 1980s and early 1990s, Soho witnessed an explosion of commercial venues which cater for a predominantly gay clientèle: bars, clubs and cafés; clothing and accessory stores; hairstylists; sex and bookshops and even a gay taxi firm. It is frequented by a predominantly white, young, affluent and fashionable group of gay men.

References

ADKINS, L. (1992) 'Sexual work and the employment of women in the service industries', in M. SAVAGE and A. WITZ (Eds) *Gender and Bureaucracy*, Oxford: Blackwell.
ALLGEIER, E. (1984) 'The personal perils of sex researchers: Vern Bulloughs and William Masters', *SIECUS Reports*, **12**, 4, pp. 16–19.

ALTMAN, D. (1986) *AIDS and the New Puritanism*, London: Pluto Press.

ALTMAN, D. (1993) 'Expertise, legitimacy and the centrality of community', in P. AGGLETON, P. DAVIES and G. HART (Eds) *AIDS: Facing The Second Decade*, London: Falmer Press.

ALTMAN, D. (1994) *Power and Community: Organizational and Cultural Responses to AIDS*, London: Taylor & Francis.

BOY GEORGE WITH BRIGHT, S. (1995) *Take It Like A Man: The Autobiography of Boy George*, London: Sidgwick & Jackson.

BRODSKY, A. (1989) 'Sex between patient and therapist: psychology's data and response', in G. O'GABBARD (Ed.) *Sexual Exploitation in Professional Relationships*, Washington DC: American Psychiatric Press.

BURRELL, G. (1984) 'Sex and organisational analysis', *Organisation Studies*, **5**, 2, pp. 97–118.

CAIN, R. (1994) 'Managing impressions of an AIDS service organization: into the mainstream or out of the closet?', *Qualitative Sociology*, **17**, 1, pp. 43–61.

Collins English Dictionary (1990) London: Collins.

CRUIKSHANK, J. (1989) 'Burnout: an issue among Canadian community development workers', *Community Development Journal*, **24**, 1, pp. 40–54.

DEVERELL, K. and PROUT, A. (1995) 'Sexuality, identity and community – the experience of MESMAC', in P. AGGLETON, P. DAVIES and G. HART (Eds) *AIDS: Safety, Sexuality and Risk*, London: Taylor & Francis.

DOCKRELL, M. (1993) 'Cum with rubbers!' in *F***sheet*, **2**, November, p. 1.

FISHER, T.D. (1989) 'Confessions of a closet sex researcher', *Journal of Sex Research*, **26**, 1, pp. 144–7.

GECHTMAN, L. (1989) 'Sexual contact between social workers and their clients', in G. O'GABBARD (Ed.) *Sexual Exploitation in Professional Relationships*, Washington DC: American Psychiatric Press.

GRIFFITHS, A. (1995) 'Services for gay men', *Agenda*, June–August, pp. 6–7.

HARRISON, T. (1995) 'Gay men and sexual health', *Agenda*, March–May, p. 5.

HEARN, J. and PARKIN, W. (1987) *Sex at Work: the Power and Paradox of Organisation Sexuality*, Brighton: Wheatsheaf Books.

HEARN, J., SHEPPARD, D.L., TANCRED-SHERIFF, P. and Burrell, G. (Eds) (1989) *The Sexuality of Organisation*, London: Sage.

HOCHSCHILD, A. (1983) *The Managed Heart: the Commercialisation of Human Feeling*, Berkeley: University of California Press.

ISHIGURO, K. (1990) *The Remains of the Day*, London: Faber & Faber.

KENNETT, S. (1995) 'Negative closets', *Capital Gay*, 3 March.

KING, E. (1993a) *Safety in Numbers*, London: Cassell.

KING, E. (1993b) 'Beating boundaries', *The Pink Paper*, 17 September.

KING, E. (1995) 'Trust the experts', *The Pink Paper*, 31 March.

LARSON, M.S. (1977) *The Rise of Professionalism*, London: University of California Press.

MACDONALD, K. (n.d.) *Professional Project and Cultural Context*, Occasional Papers in Sociology and Social Research, No.1, Guildford: Department of Sociology, University of Surrey.

MACDONALD, K. (1995) *The Sociology of the Professions*, London: Sage.

McNESTRY, M. and HARTLEY, M. (1995) *Developing a Local Response: Gay and Bisexual Men's Needs in Relation to HIV and AIDS*, London: Bexley and Greenwich Health.

O'GABBARD, G. (1989) *Sexual Exploitation in Professional Relationships*, Washington DC: American Psychiatric Press.

PARKIN, W. and GREEN, L. (1994) 'Sexuality and residential care', paper given to British Sociological Association Conference, University of Central Lancashire, 28–31 March.

PATTON, C. (1990) *Inventing AIDS*, London: Routledge.

PRINGLE, R. (1988) *Secretaries Talk: Sexuality, Power and Work*, London: Verso.

PROUT, A. and DEVERELL, K. (1995) *Working with Diversity: Building Communities, Evaluating the MESMAC Project*, London: Health Education Authority.

RUTTER, P. (1991) *Sex in the Forbidden Zone: When Men in Power – Therapists, Doctors, Clergy, Teachers and Others – Betray Women's Trust*, London: Mandala Press.

SANDFORT, T. (1995) 'HIV/AIDS prevention and the impact of attitudes toward homosexuality and bisexuality', in G. HEREK and B. GREENE (Eds) *AIDS, Identity and Community: The HIV Epidemic and Lesbians and Gay Men*, London: Sage.

SELF, W. (1993) *Cock and Bull*, London: Penguin.

STAR, L. (1989) 'The sociology of the invisible: the primacy of Anselm Strauss', in D.R. MAINES (Ed) *Social Organisation and Social Processes: Essays in Honor of Anselm Strauss*. Berlin: Aldine de Gruyter.

Time Out (1995) Talking Hearts Column, **1311**, 4–11 October, p. 158.

VANCE, C. (1991) 'Anthropology rediscovers sexuality: a theoretical comment', *Social Science and Medicine*, **33**, 8, pp. 875–84.

WEEKS, J. (1995) *Invented Moralities: Sexual Values in an Age of Uncertainty*, Oxford: Polity Press.

WEEKS, J., TAYLOR-LAYBOURN, A. and AGGLETON, P. (1994) 'An anatomy of the HIV/ AIDS voluntary sector in Britain', in P. AGGLETON, P. DAVIES and G. HART (Eds) *AIDS: Foundations for the Future*, London: Taylor & Francis.

WILLIAMS, J. (1993) 'What is a profession? Experience versus expertise', in J. WALMSLEY, J. REYNOLDS, P. SHAKESPEARE and R. WOOLFE (Eds) *Health, Welfare and Practice: Reflecting on Roles and Relationships*, London: OUP/Sage.

WILLIAMS, L. (1994) 'Front bottoms at Brighton's bushes', in *F***sheet*, **11**, p. 7.

Chapter 11

Towards Targeted HIV Prevention: An Ethnographic Study of Young Gay Men in London

Krista Maxwell

It has been argued in recent years that younger gay men may be increasingly and disproportionately at risk of HIV infection. Although previous research has investigated the attitudes of gay men generally, and of young people (usually implicitly assumed to be heterosexual), towards HIV and safer sex, relatively little attention has focused on young gay men as a group. Several studies in the US have investigated unsafe sex among young gay men (Hays, Kegeles and Coates, 1990, 1991, 1992); Hays, Kegeles and Coates claim that their results further confirm the findings of other American studies, that there is evidence of a correlation between younger age and greater 'sexual risk-taking' among gay men. Various factors are suggested as contributive: younger men in the early stages of 'coming out' may not be fully gay-identified and therefore not perceive themselves to be in a 'risk group'; negotiation of safer sex may be hampered by a lack of social skills caused by inexperience in interpersonal relationships; the young may have heightened feelings of invulnerability to risk; and younger men may perceive AIDS to be a problem of older men.

In Britain, the results of Project SIGMA's (Davies *et al.*, 1992) study do not support the contention that young gay men are at greater risk of HIV infection through unsafe sexual behaviour. Taking the number of penetrative sexual partners to be 'the most accurate indicator of risk behaviour' (*ibid.*, p. 266), they find that this factor closely resembles that of their older respondents. With regards to condom usage, they report that despite an increased incidence of anal sex among younger gay men, they are more likely to use a condom for both insertive and receptive anal intercourse. This finding is interpreted as indicative of an 'emergent culture of condom use among this generation' (*ibid.*, p. 270). Finally, knowledge of HIV and safer sex among the younger men studied was found to be at least equivalent to that of older gay men.

Davies *et al.* have criticized both the ideological bases and the methodologies of the US studies described above. They cite wide discrepancies in the employed definitions of 'young' (inter-study variations in the ceiling age range from 18 to 30), and challenge the widely drawn conclusion that 'young people in general are more likely to engage in risky behaviour than other groups' (*ibid.*, p. 260), given that the data on the 'other groups' being compared is often drawn from other studies, featuring fundamental differences in sampling design, research methodology, definitions of 'safe' and 'unsafe' sex, and definitions of 'sexual partner'. Beyond methodological considerations, Davies *et al.* express concern at what they perceive to be the generation and reinforcement of largely unsubstantiated tenets, which stigmatize and pathologize young gay men (and young people generally) as intrinsically irresponsible, socially incompetent and subject to delusions of invulnerability. Similar concerns have been voiced by Aggleton (1992, p. 81):

> In the burgeoning literature on young people and HIV/AIDS, adolescents are most frequently constructed as 'unknowledgeable', 'over pressured', 'developmentally immature', 'tragic', or 'at high risk' . . . [this construction] succeeds in homogenising and pathologising young people's experience.

Justification of HIV-prevention initiatives targeting young gay men should not need to be founded on evidence that they are at *greater* risk than older men; it should be sufficient to acknowledge that they are at risk. Whatever their relative risk of infection, it is important to appreciate that for younger men, in particular those who are just coming out, health promotion around safer sex will probably require an approach distinct to that which has been taken to date with older gay men. Fundamentally, interventions aimed at behavioural change are likely to be inappropriate for targeting behaviour which is just being initiated. Successful targeting of younger men will require a greater understanding of the unique social and emotional contexts within which young gay men are having sex; unsubstantiated clichés about the 'nature' of youth are of little value.

Various researchers and commentators concerned with the sexual behaviour of gay men in relation to HIV-prevention have expressed a felt need for more qualitative data, which might elucidate valuable information about people's own sexual identities, needs, categories and values. Ingham, Woodcock and Stenner (1992, p. 171) have called for

> a shift away from an obsession with individual knowledge or attitude scores on questionnaires towards the elucidation of meanings, powers, liabilities and constraints, from simple concepts of illness avoidance towards an acknowledgement of the importance of social reputations, and from crude frequencies towards the dynamic processes involved in creating and maintaining identities.

Where investigations are targeting younger gay men, this may be seen to be a particularly pressing need, given their relatively marginalized and disempowered position. Thus it may be argued that in this case, there is an imperative for authoritative research to accord maximum value to subjects' own words, interpretations and perspectives.

This chapter reports on research undertaken with the intention of addressing the dearth of information about the context and meaning of sexual activity, whether safe or unsafe, for young gay men. Given the evidence that young gay men in London continue to be at risk of HIV infection, and the paucity both of initiatives targeting young gay men and of information on which to base such initiatives, the investigation had two main aims. The first was to compile baseline data on sexual attitudes and behaviour of a sample of young gay men (aged under 26) in London, and to gather related quantifiable information about identity, socializing and sex education. The second aim was to use qualitative methods to learn more about young gay men's experiences and views, and thus begin to elucidate the social and cultural contexts in which attitudes to safer sex are developed. Thus the investigation had two main components: a questionnaire survey and a series of semi-structured individual interviews. This chapter concentrates on findings from the latter, although some references to data from the questionnaire survey results will be made.

Questionnaire Survey

Data were collected via self-administered questionnaires. The questionnaire included an introductory paragraph which explained the purposes of the study and gave an assurance of complete confidentiality. Postage pre-paid envelopes were provided for the return of the completed questionnaires. These were nine A4 sides in length and included the following topics: demographic details; gay identity, including involvement in the gay scene, friends' sexual identities, being out as gay/bisexual, ages first aware of gay feelings and gay identity; sexual behaviour, including relationship status, number of sexual partners and penetrative sexual partners, and gender of partners; condom use, including circumstances of use, attitudes to condoms, brands used and where condoms are obtained; relationships with people with HIV and AIDS; HIV testing; perceived risk of HIV infection; other STDs; recreational drug and alcohol use; attitudes to safer sex; sex education at school; and sources of information about safer sex. The questions relating to attitude utilized numerical response scales. Virtually all of the questions were closed with the exception of three questionnaires at the end, which asked about the personal meanings given to safer sex, opinions about which sexual practices are unsafe and the needs satisfied by sex.

The questionnaire was piloted through one gay youth group and several friends and acquaintances of the researcher. The final draft was also discussed in some detail with a focus group of young gay men conducted at the youth group. Two hundred and forty-five copies of the final version were distributed through gay youth groups, gay societies at universities and colleges, gay clubs and bars, and friends and acquaintances of people reached through the above network, and of the researcher. It is hoped that the use of 'snowballing' as a recruitment technique may have helped to increase the representativeness of the sample. The target group was defined as including young men under the age of 26, who identified themselves as gay, bisexual and/or having sex with men, and who lived and/or socialized in London. Returned questionnaires not meeting these criteria were not included in the results.

Sixty-nine of the returned questionnaires were included in the study, and it was decided to further include seven questionnaires from the final stage of the pilot study, making a total of 76 questionnaires which were included in the final analysis. It was not possible to calculate an accurate response rate, as it is known that not all questionnaires distributed via social groups were handed out to individuals, and some groups took the initiative of photocopying questionnaires for further distribution when they ran low. The returned questionnaires were allocated code numbers, and the data was analysed using Epi Info[1] (version 5.01b, July 1991).

Interviews

The qualitative phase of the study involved in-depth interviews, some informal interviews and 'participant observation' (necessarily limited) in gay clubs, bars and youth groups. Interview subjects were mostly recruited via the questionnaire: respondents were asked if they would be willing to participate in an interview to further discuss the issues raised by the questionnaire. Those interested were given the option of either writing a contact telephone number on the questionnaire, contacting the researcher directly at a telephone number which was provided, or (if they had received the questionnaire through a youth group) organizing the interview through a youth worker. An unexpectedly large proportion of respondents (46 per cent) indicated a willingness to be interviewed; unfortunately time constraints meant that not all of these were interviewed. A few interviews were also arranged in person, through friends and acquaintances, and with young men spoken to in nightclubs. In all cases, the interviewee was encouraged to choose the place of interview: either his home or workplace, a private room at a youth group's meeting place, or a private flat arranged by the interviewer. Interviews were conducted over a period of two months with fifteen different young men (two of whom were interviewed twice), who were offered a small cash payment to cover expenses.

All of those interviewed had also completed questionnaires. The fifteen young gay and bisexual men interviewed represented a broad spectrum of experience. They ranged in age from 17 to 25, although the majority of those interviewed were under age 21. Some had only come out in recent months, others had been out for several years. About half were involved (to varying degrees) in gay youth groups. Subjects also varied in terms of nationality, occupation, ethnicity and social class.

Of seventeen interviews, seven were conducted at the home of the interviewee, seven at private flats arranged by the interviewer, two at the interviewee's workplace, and one at a youth club. All interviews were one-on-one and conducted in complete privacy. They averaged about two hours in length. The interviews were semi-structured, the interviewer introducing various questions and themes, and the interviewee was encouraged to introduce any topics he felt to be relevant. The interviews also included discussion of safer sex promotional material introduced by the interviewer: Gay Men Fighting AIDS (GMFA) postcards, and the Terence Higgins Trust's small photo-comic-strip leaflets, which depict gay men in various situations involving the practice of safer sex. All the interviews were tape-recorded and later transcribed.

Selected Results from Questionnaire Survey

Table 11.1 provides some sociodemographic data describing the two samples: those responding to the questionnaire survey (respondents), and those taking part in interviews (informants). The latter group is subsumed within the former. The two groups show broadly similar characteristics, although the interview sample included a slightly higher proportion of men who were unemployed (perhaps because these men may have had more free time in which to be interviewed) and had reached a higher level of education. The interview sample also contained a slightly higher proportion of African and Afro–Caribbean men than the questionnaire sample, and a slightly higher proportion of those identifying themselves as bisexual or 'other', rather than gay.

Tables 11.2, 11.3 and 11.4 provide information about respondents' sexual identities and social lives. The ages at which respondents report having first been aware of gay feelings fall within a very large range, as do the ages at which respondents report having first identified themselves as gay. The difference between the mean ages for the two questions is nearly four-and-a-half years. Table 11.3 shows what proportion of respondents' friends identify as gay, with a comparison of responses from older and younger respondents. Respondents under the age of 21 are significantly more likely to report that less than half of their friends identify as gay ($x^2 = 9.24$, df = 2, $p < 0.01$). Similarly, Table 11.4 shows that the younger respondents are less likely to describe the context of their social life as mainly gay, and more likely to describe it as both gay and straight.

Table 11.1 *Selected Results from Questionnaire Survey*

Characteristics of samples	Respondents (n = 76)	Informants (n = 15)
Age		
Mean	21	20.8
Range	16–25	17–25
Employment		
Student	46%	33%
Employed full-time	30%	26%
Employed part-time	13%	13%
Unemployed	16%	26%
Highest level of educational achievement		
GCSE/O levels	18%	20%
A levels/BTEC/Diploma	51%	53%
Degree or higher	20%	26%
Nationality (n = 75)		
British	75%	66%
Other European	15%	26%
Other	10%	7%
Self-identified ethnic group (n = 73)		
White/European	85%	86%
Afro-Caribbean	5%	10%
South Asian	4%	–
African	3%	4%
Chinese/Japanese	3%	–
Self-identified sexual orientation		
Gay	87%	80%
Bisexual	10%	13%
Other	3%	7%

Table 11.2 *Gay identity and social life*

Age of first gay feelings/identity

	Mean	Range
Age first aware of gay feelings (n = 71)	10.2	3–20
Age first identified as gay/ put a label to gay feelings (n = 71)	14.7	7–22

175

Table 11.3 *Number of friends identifying as gay*

	Under 21 (n = 34)	21 and older (n = 42)
All	–	10%
More than half	21%	40%
Roughly half	35%	36%
Less than half	38%	14%
None	6%	–

Table 11.4 *Context of social life*

	Aged under 21 (n = 34)	Aged 21 and older (n = 42)
Gay	21%	48%
Straight	9%	5%
Both	68%	45%
Neither	3%	2%

Interview Results

The following excerpts from interviews with young gay men have been selected as representative of some of the major issues which emerged from the interview material, and should serve to provide some insight into the nature of these young gay men's early sociosexual experiences. Names have been changed to protect informants' identities.

Gay Identity, Pre-scene

In response to questions about when they first felt themselves to be gay, some informants indicated that they had been aware of their gay status since early adolescence, or even earlier.

> My first gay experience was when I was twelve. I *knew* I was gay then. You hear MPs saying that it's an experiment, or a phase . . . I *knew.* (Paul, age 17)

> I. Was there a point when you suddenly thought, 'I'm gay'?

> Yeah, it must have been when I was about thirteen . . . I realized, like, yeah I'm gay. Oh, well. But I never did anything about it, I didn't tell anyone. I went to a Catholic school, lots of nuns there, so, not a good idea. (Jake, age 20)

I've always known, ever since I was small. I remember walking down the street with my friend, I must have been under seven, and I remember saying to her, 'Do you like big men?' or something, and she goes, 'No!' So I said, 'Neither do I.' But I did, I wanted to say yes. I've always known that I liked men instead of women. I did have a girlfriend when I was about twelve, but it's just something that I did because all my friends were doing it, it didn't mean anything. (David, age 19)

Others reported having been less confident of their gay feelings and identity, and participated in gay sex and gay relationships without identifying as gay, either overtly or to themselves.

Some people actually come out, and then they go out and have their relationships or whatever. I suddenly found myself in this relationship, and it was only a while after I'd been going out with him, I guess I labelled myself as bisexual as sort of a cop-out to begin with . . . After splitting up with G., a state of confusion set in. I didn't want to go to gay places at all, I think it was another six months after we split up before I went to a gay place. I had six months of celibacy, and it was only then that I began to think, am I gay? Am I bisexual? Why am I attracted to men? Is it just G., are there going to be other men I'm attracted to? That was the roughest time I've ever had. (Martin, age 24)

I think I was first attracted to men around thirteen, fourteen . . . at the time I was really confused 'cause I also felt a general attraction to women. Although I'd had sex with men, I didn't realize I was gay until I'd said it to somebody else, and that was when I was sixteen . . . I suddenly sat back and thought, my god, I've been gay for like, years! (Scott, age 17)

Sex and Relationships, Pre-scene

Informants described a range of experiences of sexual relationships with other men, in the days before they had come out on the gay scene. Some reported having had sex with other young men of similar ages to themselves, while others were involved with older men: someone met at work, through the classified section of a gay paper, and in one case the stepfather of a young woman with whom the informant was having a relationship. Informants described some instances in which condoms had been used, and some in which they had had sex without condoms.

He was my brother's friend, and he was staying round my house. I was twelve, he was about fourteen or fifteen. He made the first move, but I wasn't molested or anything like that. After the first time he stayed round my house more, nearly once a week, and there was like a boyfriend sort of thing going, but not really . . . it was really just sex.

I.   And did you know anything about safer sex at the time?

Oh, no. I didn't know about how AIDS was caught or anything then. (Paul, age 17)

I was fifteen, and it was with my girlfriend's step-father that I first had sex with a man. He started coming on to me, and I ignored it, 'cause obviously he was with her mum, and had a kid with her. Until I suddenly thought, actually, I like him back ! So we started having sex in his car. He was 31. So that went on for about five or six months, then he dumped me when he found out I was sleeping with my girlfriend at the same time.

I.   Do you remember if you were very aware about safer sex at that time?

I think I was because I was sleeping with my girlfriend, so with her I was having protected sex more as a form of contraception, but also I didn't want to catch anything. (Scott, age 17)

Sex and Relationships on the Scene

Early Days on the Scene

Most informants described their first experiences of the gay scene as an emotionally intense, often overwhelming period. Some felt deeply reassured to see so many other men like themselves. For some, the experience of coming out on the scene apparently symbolized a social and often sexual acknowledgment of a hitherto unexpressed gay identity. 'It was like my first night of being gay really, my first night on the gay scene.' (David, age 19, who came out last year)

The scene often presented a first opportunity to connect with other men, emotionally and/or sexually, after what in most cases had been a relatively lonely and socially isolated adolescence:

I'd really like to be in love with somebody. If you're straight you can have girlfriends and boyfriends from a very early age, and it isn't frowned upon. But I'm nineteen now, I've just come out and it's something I'd like to experience. (Luke, age 19)

Some reported feeling a sense of urgency around gaining sexual experience: a combination of making up for lost time and, for some, being unsure of when their next opportunity to make contact with other gay men might be – as in the case of this 24-year-old (reflecting on his first night on the scene at age nineteen):

Within the hour he fixed me up with somebody at the club, a 23-year-old . . . went back to his place. I know I shouldn't have gone, 'cause you just don't know with these guys, do you, but anyway I did. Such is the pressure of being young and gay, because your experiences, you believe, are going to be so far and wide apart, that you take every opportunity you can. (Michael, age 24)

Premature Labelling of 'Relationships'

Several informants, all under 21 and relatively new to the scene, described situations in which they or a friend had become involved with a man whom they expected was going to be a regular, potentially long-term partner – only to find that the man in question had interpreted the situation differently:

I've only had one [experience of anal sex since the previous interview] . . . that was because I was really taken with Chris and he seemed to be taken with me. It was all 'wow', and it was like me being really stupid on the first night, getting into talking about, 'Oh, I want a relationship' and everything, and he said 'Oh, well, I want a relationship as well', and we decided we were going to go out, you see. And then I called him again a couple of days later – he never called me or anything – and his flatmate said, 'Oh, he's not in, but he told me to tell you not to bother calling here again.' And I was so hurt. (Liam, age 19)

Evolving Attitudes

Reports from slightly older or more experienced informants indicate that they too were preoccupied with finding a 'relationship' in their earlier days on the scene. However, it seems that most abandon this goal – at least outwardly – as they gain more experience of the sexual dynamics of the gay scene.

> Towards relationships, [when he was younger] I was thinking, yeah,
> I'll have a relationship, but I've tried it and it doesn't work...
> I don't like people telling me what to do, or relying on me to do
> anything. Now I'm laidback. But then I was like, a bit uptight, stuff
> like that. (Jake, age 20)

> When you are young, you dream about these romantic relationships
> in which you're going to do anything for your boyfriend ... but then
> because of what you see happening, you start to become selfish ... and
> it's happening to me, and I've seen it happening to other people –
> they don't look for a relationship any more. (Roland, age 22)

The more experienced informants also expressed feeling more in control
of their destiny on the scene, in contrast to their younger selves, whom they
often characterized as vulnerable to the whims of other, usually older, men
on the scene:

> When you're younger, if you're not so sorted out inside, then I'd say
> you want a relationship. You see a lot of sixteen-year-olds who are
> like, always with 30-year-olds, 40-year-olds ... they haven't quite figured
> out what's happening. They're just looking for someone to tell them
> it's OK to be gay. But then when you figure out what's happening on
> the scene and everything, you've got your own choice, you do what
> you want. (Jake, age 20)

> Back then, I really just slept with the first people who came up to me.
> It's not that I was some young, incredibly attractive person, it's just
> that I was some young incredibly *stupid* person, who slept with any-
> one who came on to me. (Scott, age 17)

Unprotected Sex in Relationships

Although both the questionnaire sample and the interview sample demonstrated themselves to be largely well-informed about safer sex, and to have
condom-friendly attitudes, a large minority of both groups reported not always
using condoms. Comments made by informants serve to illustrate the possible
motivations behind choosing to have unprotected sex:

> Condoms aren't intimate ... they break the atmosphere between
> us. (Mark, age 24)

> It sort of seems more real when there's not that little bit of
> rubber between you ... it sort of seems that there's more of a

relationship there if you can [have sex without a condom]. (Paul, age 17)

I know about people who go into a relationship, and after they've been together one month, they stop using condoms and so on. I think it's silly . . . [but] obviously the temptation is quite big, 'cause you feel, I want to be different to the others, so I'll give him something special, which is my body in an unsafe way. (Roland, age 22)

I. So can you imagine that if you were in a longer-term relationship, you might want to stop using them [condoms]?

Yeah, I think I probably would. I don't know how you would go about getting tests, but I think we should ask if we could both have tests. If that relationship is getting on quite well, then I'd trust him not to have sex with anybody else.

I. How long do you think you would wait in a relationship before you would stop using them?

A few weeks, then I'd persuade him to have a test . . . I think it's four weeks until your results come through. I don't know, I've never had a long-term relationship like that. (Paul, age 17)

Young Gay Men and Friendship

It emerged from the interviews that most of the informants had experienced friendship between young gay men as often highly problematic, and most had failed to form or maintain many or any close friendships with other young gay men. Various possible explanations for this were suggested, including a pervasive superficiality and over-emphasis on sex that some informants claimed were features of the gay scene:

I've found young gay men very superficial. I mean I've been meeting lots and lots of people, and I can tell you that I have very few close friends. And that's why I feel that lots of gay guys are very lonely, especially the young ones. I think that there are very few close friendships. (Roland, age 22)

It's a lot harder to be friends with gay men. I mean there's no respect between gay men, I don't know why it is . . . you can't be

181

really *close* friends, you can't tell them everything. 'Cause it's like, 'Oh, you slut!' or 'You didn't!' or whatever. They pass judgement, a lot of gay men do pass judgement on other gay men. (Jake, age 20)

I've always found that really strange, I've never really made any friends in gay places . . . I've found, they just want to get you into bed, and then they don't want to know you any more. (Carl, age 18)

Many informants, particularly those at the younger end of the sample range, reported having close relationships with young women (usually heterosexual, but occasionally lesbian):

I prefer being friends with girls, anyway. I have maybe two really close friends, both women, one's a lesbian and one's straight. (Jake, age 20)

Most of them are girls, actually, that I've told [that I'm gay]. We are quite close, especially me and one girl. She's very liberal, and I decided I'd tell her, 'cause whenever anyone ever slagged off a Black person or a gay person, you know like 'queers, dirty ass', whatever they say, then you know, she'd sort of put them in their place. So I told her. We're sort of best friends now. (Paul, age 17)

That was the roughest time I've ever had [coming out]. I had some quite close [female] friends . . . one in particular, Alice was very, very open-minded, and experienced in all sorts of issues herself, so she was able to offer me consolation and also useful advice. So she was the person I talked to most of all. (Martin, age 24)

Discussion

All the questionnaire and interview respondents identified as either gay, bisexual or somewhere in between. Beyond these characteristics, it would be inaccurate to construe the sample as a homogeneous group. However, some level of involvement in the gay scene is a prominent common factor. To the extent that the results of this study can be taken as representative of a 'group', I therefore suggest that they may reflect some of the attitudes and behaviours of young gay men involved in the commercial gay scene in London.

The London gay scene has played a significant role in the lives of all of the young gay men interviewed, if not at the time of interview then at some time in the recent past. Data from the questionnaire survey suggests that involvement in the scene features in the lives of virtually all respondents:

60 per cent report regularly going to gay venues, and a further 34 per cent occasionally do so. Indeed, there are few other options available to young gay men looking for friends and boyfriends. Although gay youth groups, where they exist, often present themselves as an alternative to the commercial scene, survey respondents mentioning youth-group membership also usually attend commercial venues (although several of those interviewed who were youth-group members reported that a small number of other group members are not involved in the scene at all).

Early Gay Experience: Gay Identity, Sex and Relationships, Pre-scene

Given the apparently significant influence of the gay scene on the attitudes and experiences of those interviewed, it is important to make a distinction between relationships conducted during a 'pre-scene' period, and those occurring after a young man has come on the scene. This is not to imply that there is an inevitability of gay experiences leading to involvement in the scene, although this has clearly been the pattern for those interviewed in the current study. It seems reasonable to assume that there are other young men having sex with men who, for whatever reasons, may never become involved with the scene, nor with any organized gay social life. This assumption is supported by reports from several interviewees who described early sexual experiences with other young men, whom they know not to be currently involved in the gay scene or gay social groups, nor to have assumed any overt gay identity. As an illustration, one seventeen-year-old respondent reported having regularly had sexual encounters with 'straight' young men in the toilets at 'straight' raves.

Gay Identity, Pre-scene

Many young men in this 'pre-scene' stage have a strong sense of their sexual orientation and identity from a young age, as evidenced both by personal accounts, and from questionnaire-survey results: the mean reported age of first awareness of gay feelings is 10.2, and the mean reported age of first self-identifying as gay is 14.7. The mean age of first experience of anal sex is 17.8, but the range here is large (8–24). The interview findings indicate that some young men may not identify themselves as gay until after they have been involved in gay sex and relationships and, in several cases, the respondent's first gay sexual encounter was with an equally non-gay-identified individual.

Clearly, accessing young men who are behaviourally homosexual, are not involved in any organized gay social life, and may or may not identify themselves as gay, poses particular problems both for research and health promotion. Personal histories provided by informants about their 'pre-scene' days (in some cases very recent), give some insight into the nature of young gay experience outside the scene. It appears highly variable in terms of age of partner, sexual practice, the level of the subject's awareness of safer sex, and whether safer or unsafe sex is practised. However, a factor apparently common to most of the encounters described by informants is that *neither* partner is gay-identified. Scott (1993) has asserted that 'even those MWHSWM who identify themselves as heterosexual will, in practice, have sexual encounters with confident gay and bisexual men', and goes on to argue that such out gay or bisexual men are the most effective means of influencing men 'on the margins' of gay social scenes. On the basis of this assumption, King (1993, p. 205) has described such encounters as 'the most efficient form of safer sex peer education' for reaching non-gay identified men who have sex with men. The above accounts illustrate that in the case of young gay men not on the scene, such sexual contact with 'confident' gay men can clearly not be relied on as a source of safer sex education.

Sex and Relationships on the Scene: Early Days and Evolving Attitudes

In retrospect many informants felt that, having not come out until their late teens in most cases, they were deprived of a true adolescence. At a stage when most heterosexual young people are experimenting with relationships and sexuality, most young gay men are isolated from potential boyfriends, with little or no means of sexual self-expression available to them. As Plummer (1989, p. 208) has pointed out:

> [for heterosexual young people] schools, youth clubs and the work-place become key locations for finding boyfriends and girlfriends. In contrast, for gay young people, these places are highly alienating as they constantly reinforce their difference and provide no pathways to partners or relevant experience.

Thus when they do come out on to the scene, go to a gay club for the first time and are suddenly in contact with lots of potential sexual partners, it is hardly surprising that many feel a need to make up for lost time. Being presented with opportunities for sexual contact in an environment which is not repressing and condemning their sexuality, but actively encouraging it, creates a situation which many respondents described in terms of a rite of passage, symbolizing the beginning of their gay identity. For most young gay men, their experience of coming out on the scene is seen as their first opportunity for a relationship. Thus most informants described feeling a deep yearning to be close to someone, emotionally and/or sexually; for young gay men, this desire has an added intensity stemming from years of social and sexual isolation and repression. Evidently, a young gay man's early days on the scene often constitute a highly charged period, laden with emotional expectation.

From the time when they first start getting involved in the scene, many young gay men undergo a characteristic evolution of their attitudes to sex and relationships. One aspect of this evolution involves a less overt interest in achieving a long-term relationship, often accompanied by an increasing acceptance or justification of (or resignation to) long-term promiscuity. Another aspect of this transition involves issues of empowerment and control. In retrospect, some informants characterized their younger selves, new to the scene, as naïve, vulnerable, hopelessly idealistic. They felt scornful towards what they now perceive to have been a complete lack of awareness and discernment. A few informants reported that developing a familiarity with the scene, and an awareness of the dynamics of sex on the scene, has given them a sense of control, of being able to pursue their own sexual interests and refuse unwanted advances. In contrast, others report that their increasing experience of the scene has only served to underline their inherent powerlessness: ultimately, they feel, older men will always have the upper hand.

Sex and Relationships on the Scene: Premature Labelling of 'Relationships'

Davies *et al.* (1992) have found that young gay men (under 21 years) are more likely to report being in regular sexual relationships, when compared to older gay men in their cohort, and speculate that this difference may indicate 'a specific response to AIDS or a more embedded feature of the sexual career' (Davies *et al.*, 1992, p. 269). I suggest that this difference may also be attributable to the tendency of younger men, especially those in the earlier stages of coming out, to romanticize and idealize their sexual encounters, such that an encounter (or brief series of encounters) which a more experienced person would recognize and classify as casual or a one-off, is perceived to be the early stages of a committed, long-term relationship. A tendency to repeatedly rush into labelling a sexual encounter as a relationship may be seen as a natural response to the situation most young gay men just coming out on the scene find themselves in: feeling an intense need for intimacy often after years of emotional isolation, wanting to validate their previously suppressed sexuality and being suddenly overwhelmed by a large number of potential sexual partners. Holland *et al.* (1992, p. 281) have observed a similar tendency in young women who may define sexual encounters as 'steady, despite objective circumstances'. They report that young women experience:

> social pressure to define their relationships as steady. The term casual has negative connotations so that very few describe themselves as having such relations. Steady relationships were defined as those based on trust and/or love, criteria which had little to do with temporality and less to do with the practice of safer sex.

Young gay men growing up in this society are generally no less susceptible to cultural influences which idealize and romanticize the notion of (heterosexual) monogamy. In the absence of alternative value systems, it is not surprising that many will come on to the scene with a gay version of this ideal in mind: as one seventeen-year-old informant expressed it, 'like a husband and wife relationship but with two husbands'. The ideal of monogamy has been further promoted by many health-education messages (generally aimed at populations assumed to be homogeneously heterosexual) as a strategy for HIV-prevention. As King (1993, p. 147) has pointed out, despite the possible value of such a strategy for those 'having unprotected sex in a low-prevalence environment, such as the vast majority of heterosexuals in Britain', this message may have ominous consequences for a gay man having sex in a high-prevalence context such as the current London scene.

Sex and Relationships on the Scene: Unsafe Sex in Relationships

Recent data from studies in the US and the UK has indicated that most unprotected anal sex between gay men is taking place within the contexts of relationships (Hays, Kegeles and Coates, 1990, 1991, 1992; Davies *et al.*, 1993). As Davies *et al.* (1992, p. 269) have pointed out, where unprotected sex within a relationship is initiated 'before strictly epidemiological considerations would dictate', monogamy as an attempt at minimizing the risk of infection is of dubious efficacy. Sex within a relationship after both partners have tested negative may only be considered safe where (1) both tests were timed so as to avoid the risk of false negatives, i.e. sufficient time allowed after any possible previous exposure to infection for antibodies to develop (three months is usually recommended as the minimum); (2) both partners have been practising exclusively safe sex in this period; and (3) neither partner has engaged in any subsequent risky behaviour.

Results from both the questionnaire survey and interviews with respondents indicate that being in a relationship may be strongly associated with the practice of unprotected sex by some young gay men. This association may be of particular concern, given the observed tendency of younger men towards the premature labelling of 'relationships'. Furthermore, comments made by a few respondents illustrate that at least some young gay men may have a poor understanding of the time lag between HIV infection and the ability of tests to detect such infection.

Prieur (1990, p. 113) has observed that 'Accepting semen has been an important value in the gay culture, a way of showing devotion and belonging'. She emphasizes the value of sex as communication within a close relationship and suggests that 'In this communication, a condom is a negative message, and refusing the semen is a rejection.' Levine and Siegel (1992) have documented various cases of gay men explaining occurrences of unsafe sex as demonstrations of feeling towards their partners. Some have 'described their behaviour as a sacrifice made for their partners, which was attributable to understandable and even altruistic motives' (*ibid.*, p. 63). The results of this study indicate that such interpretations are valid for some young gay men in relationships – or in what they hope will become a relationship. In response to the statement, 'In a serious relationship, having sex without a condom can express intimacy and trust in one another,' 40 per cent of respondents expressed agreement or strong agreement. Comments made by informants during interviews further confirm that young gay men see unprotected sex within the context of a perceived relationship as highly significant.

Early experiences of gay sex on the scene are often of great significance, not only in terms of being the first opportunity for intimacy following years of isolation, but also as a physical validation of a young gay man's sexual identity: up to that point, an identity subject to denial, stigmatization and derision. Young gay men in relationships may be tempted to stop using condoms in order to signify the permanence of the relationship, to demonstrate trust in their partner or to achieve a sense of greater intimacy. An appreciation of the many layers of significance of early sexual experience may facilitate an understanding of why some young gay men may choose not to use condoms at this stage of their sexual career.

Young Gay Men and Friendship

Many respondents reported that they had experienced difficulties in sustaining friendships with other young gay men. This was particularly the case for the younger men, those who had come out most recently and those who were very involved in the club scene. Many felt that close friendships between young gay men are inherently problematic and suggested various reasons for this. A frequent reference was sex 'getting in the way' of friendship: sexual competition and jealousy; two friends having sex and then finding that destroyed their friendship; or one friend being attracted to the other and finding his feelings not reciprocated. Many respondents complained of a general superficiality, bitchiness and lack of trust pervading in the gay scene, creating a social climate which makes keeping friends difficult.

Close friendships with young women (usually straight but sometimes lesbian) played a prominent role in the lives of almost all respondents. These were often described as featuring a stability and level of trust less common in friendships between young gay men. In almost every case, respondents reported coming out to a close female friend before anyone else, and receiving a lot of support from female friends during this usually difficult period. Most of those interviewed expressed a strong preference for mixed rather than men-only clubs, the exceptions being a couple of older informants (24 and 25 years old), who reported that they preferred men-only clubs because 'there's more to choose from'. However, one of them added that when he first came out, he had had a definite preference for clubs attended by women too. There are various possible explanations for this preference. First, for those just coming out and not entirely comfortable with their sexuality, the presence of women creates a more familiar environment, more evocative of 'normal' society. Second, many young gay men report feeling threatened and 'preyed upon' in men-only clubs, in which, some say, sex becomes the only focus and the atmosphere is more aggressive. In discussions about different clubs in London, the two which were repeatedly cited as the 'hardest' places are both men-only. In mixed clubs, it was felt, more people are there to enjoy themselves and socialize with friends and not necessarily to pick up. Finally, many respondents reported that their female friends enjoy going out to gay places and, given the importance of these friendships, it is not surprising that many young men would prefer places to which they can bring their female friends.

Conclusions

This study has established the beginnings of a contextualized understanding of the sociosexual lives of young gay men on the London scene. I have illustrated the significance of the scene in impacting on individuals' evolving sexual attitudes and behaviour, and suggested that it may be helpful to view young gay men's sexual 'careers' in terms of pre-scene, early scene and later scene stages.

It has been observed that many young gay men value highly the friendship of young women, while close friendships between young gay men tend often to be problematic. Within the questionnaire-survey sample, the younger men (under 21) report a significantly smaller proportion of their friends identifying as gay compared to those over 21. These findings indicate that young gay men cannot be assumed to be socializing within a context which constitutes, or even approaches, a supportive gay milieu. If peer education approaches to health promotion are based on such assumptions, they will probably be inaccessible to, and ineffective for, a majority of younger gay men, particularly teenagers. On the other hand, many young gay men seem to have a strong mutual empathy with young women and, given the relative vulnerability of both groups, it might be appropriate for health-education interventions to capitalize on this. Such a strategy might be particularly relevant to a school environment, as it has been observed that young women and gay men may tend to form close alliances in this context.

Various factors and scenarios have been identified as associated with the practice of unprotected sex by young gay men. Sexual encounters in the 'pre-scene' stage may often occur with non-gay-identified partners, thus making it likely that neither partner will have accessed safer sex publicity aimed at gay men. The tendency for younger men to prematurely label sexual encounters as 'relationships' has been discussed. This tendency is of particular significance give the evidence from elsewhere, supported by the findings of this study, that being in a relationship is frequently associated with the practice of unprotected sex. Reasons for choosing to participate in unprotected sex which have emerged as salient for some of the young gay men in this study, include signifying the permanence of a relationship and achieving a sense of greater intimacy. The significance of these meanings is best understood against the historical backdrop of young gay men's pre-scene and early scene stages.

The importance of targeting both young gay men not on the scene, and those new to the scene, cannot be over-emphasized; indeed, these two groups were frequently mentioned by respondents as being particularly in need of focused campaigns. There is a need for campaigns via mainstream channels of communication (notwithstanding the many obstacles to this presented by a homophobic society) such as the mass media and the education system, to reach young men before they come on the scene, and those marginal to the scene. Indeed, a more comprehensive and relevant sex education which begins to address the needs of young gay men (and young lesbians and bisexuals) is essential, in order to address the complex issues of empowerment and self-esteem which have been touched on, but which are clearly fundamental to the promotion of sexual health. Finally, regarding the issue of unprotected sex in relationships, I would echo Hickson *et al.* (1994) in calling for 'campaigns that recognize and respect the variety of decision-making in gay men's sex lives', via an acknowledgement of the possibility of unprotected but risk-free sex, the validity of personal strategies and the role of voluntary HIV testing.

Acknowledgments

I should like to express my gratitude to the many young men who responded to and distributed questionnaires, and to those who shared details of their lives as participants in very personal interviews and discussions. Thanks are also given to the youth group staff who helped to distribute questionnaires. David Gellner, Ford Hickson and Chris McKevitt provided much appreciated feedback on various earlier drafts of this chapter. All opinions and any errors are my own. The research on which this paper is based was undertaken for a BSc Hons dissertation at Oxford Brookes University, Oxford.

Note

1 Epi Info is designed by Dean *et al.* (1994), Centers for Disease Control and Prevention, Atlanta, Georgia, USA.

References

AGGLETON, P. (with DANKMEIJER, P.) (1992) 'Young people, sexual health and HIV/ AIDS', in H. CURTIS (Ed.) *Promoting Sexual Health*, London: BMA Foundation for AIDS.

DAVIES, P.M., HICKSON, F.C.I., WEATHERBURN, P. and HUNT, A.J. (1993) *Sex, Gay Men and AIDS*, London: Falmer Press.

DAVIES, P.M., WEATHERBURN, P., HUNT, A.J., HICKSON, F.C.I., McMANUS, T.J. and COXON, A.P.M. (1992) 'The sexual behaviour of young gay men in England and Wales', *AIDS Care*, 4, 3, pp. 259–72.

DEAN, A.G., DEAN, J.A., COULOMBIER, D., BRENDEL, K.A., SMITH, D.C., BURTON, A.H., DICKER, R.C., SULLIVAN, K., FAGAN, R.F. and ARNER, T.G. (1994) Epi Info, Version 6: a word processing, database, and statistics program for epidemiology on micro-computers. Atlanta, Georgia USA: Centers for Disease Control and Prevention.

HAYS, R.B., KEGELES, S.M. and COATES, T.J. (1990) 'High HIV risk-taking among young gay men', *AIDS*, 4, pp. 901–7.

HAYS, R.B., KEGELES, S.M. and COATES, T.J. (1991) 'Understanding the high rates of HIV risk-taking among young gay and bisexual men: the Young Men's Survey', *International Conference on AIDS* 7, 1, 16–21 June, PG 48 (abstract no. MC 101).

HAYS, R.B., KEGELES, S.M. and COATES, T.J. (1992) 'Changes in peer norms and sexual enjoyment predict changes in sexual risk-taking among young gay men', *International Conference on AIDS 8*, 2, 19–24 July, PG D417 (abstract no. POD 5183).

HICKSON, F., WEATHERBURN, P., KEOGH, P. and DAVIES, P. (1994) 'Perception of partners' HIV status and unprotected anal intercourse (UAI) among gay men', conference presentation, AIDS Impact: Second Conference of Bio-Socio-Psycho Aspects of HIV/AIDS, Brighton.

HOLLAND, J., RAMANAZOGLU, C., SCOTT, S., SHARPE, S. and THOMSON, R. (1992)

'Risk, power and the possibility of pleasure: young women and safer sex', *AIDS Care*, **4**, 3, pp. 259–72.

INGHAM, R., WOODCOCK, A. and STENNER, K. (1992) 'The limitations of rational decision-making as applied to young people's sexual behaviour', in P. AGGLETON, P. DAVIES and G. HART (Eds) *AIDS: Rights, Risk and Reason*, London: Falmer Press.

KING, E. (1993) *Safety in Numbers: Safer Sex and Gay Men*, London: Cassell.

LEVINE, C. and SIEGEL, L. (1992) 'Unprotected sex: understanding gay men's participation', in J. HUBER and B.E. SCHNEIDER (Eds) *The Social Context of AIDS*, London, Sage.

PLUMMER, K. (1989) 'Lesbian and gay youth in England', in G. HERDT (Ed.) *Gay and Lesbian Youth*, New York: Harrington Park Press.

PRIEUR, A. (1990) 'Norwegian gay men: reasons for continued practice of unsafe sex', *AIDS Education and Prevention*, **2**, 2, pp. 109–15.

SCOTT, P. (1993) 'Beginning HIV prevention work with gay and bisexual men', in B. EVANS, S. SANDBERG and S. WATSON (Eds) *Healthy Alliances in HIV Prevention*, London: Health Education Authority.

Chapter 12

Identities and Gay Men's Sexual Decision-making

Paul Flowers, Jonathan A. Smith, Paschal Sheeran and Nigel Beail

Much of the sexual health research to date has been based around the dictates of urgency rather than rigour (Catania *et al.*, 1990) or, as Bolton (1992, p. 128) puts it, 'superficiality was privileged over complexity'. Because this new interest in sexual behaviour has been fuelled by public health concerns, the resulting body of knowledge has been shaped by a largely medical conception of sex. Arguably, this medical conception also extends to understanding how people make decisions around choice of partner, choice of sexual acts and decisions relating to condom use. In this manner sexual decisions are recouched in terms of health decisions. This new field can quite accurately be described as the study of 'sexual *health*' as opposed to sexual *behaviour*. This chapter begins to describe the problematic nature of HIV-prevention work grounded solely within the sexual health paradigm.

Sexual activity has been conceptualized within the constraints of the sexual health paradigm. Epidemiology has been a central part of this process. While essential in identifying the differential risks of differing sexual acts, epidemiology has lent a distinct somatic slant to our understanding of gay men's sexual risk behaviour. This understanding, as Hart and Boulton (1995, p. 55) point out, 'does not address an entirely separate, but equally significant dimension of risk, notably how and why this occurs to particular individuals, in specific contexts and at certain times'. In other words, the commonality of shared physical behaviour (particularly anal intercourse) is assumed to reflect shared volition, agency, identity and indeed a shared community. Equally, the assumed motivations to have sex are grounded in somatic understandings of sexual activity. It is assumed that the desire for sensate pleasure dictates decisions relating to the choice of sexual acts and indeed decisions relating to condom use. In this way, among men engaging in sexual activity with other men, sexual health theory, like epidemiology, addresses the sexual act as the prime site of decisions relating to risk reduction. Costs-and-benefits analyses weigh up the loss of physical sensation (through condom use or the adoption of non-penetrative sex) with the gains of HIV risk reduction. As such, sexual health-promotion practice responds through the provision of both information about risks per act and by providing condoms, and this is understood as adequately addressing the totality of gay men's sexual health needs.

The key point of this chapter is that though epidemiology and health promotion posit sexual acts as the locus of HIV risk, if we look beyond this somatic level, it becomes clear that people perceive other, often more important indices of risk, such as identities (Spears *et al.*, 1992; Kitzinger, 1993; Waldby, Kippax and Crawford, 1993; Wight, 1993).

Work which is not entrenched within the sexual health paradigm is particularly useful as it can provide a contextualized account of the relationship between sexual behaviour and sexual health. For example, the studies of Prieur (1990), Dowsett, Davis and Connell (1992) and Boulton *et al.* (1995), provide qualitative data which add depth and insight to our understanding of quantitative findings and clearly illustrate participants' understandings of issues.

The study reported in this chapter explores the relationship between sexual health and identities in its broadest sense. It does not assume to know *a priori* the salient beliefs about sexual identity and its relation to sexual behaviour. Instead, this study employed a form of grounded theory (Glaser and Strauss, 1967) to describe and explore those beliefs. Rather than addressing particular hypotheses or detailed research questions, the study takes men's accounts of this relationship as its prime focus. However, before examining men's understandings of the links between identity and sexual behaviour it is worth looking at the existing literature.

Sexual identity and particularly gay identity have been central in the history of fighting the HIV and AIDS epidemic. Gay men invented safer sex (Callen, 1983) and in the face of continuing state reticence (Shilts, 1987; King, 1993) gay men continue to produce some of the most dynamic and direct sexual health promotion (for example, in the UK, through Gay Men Fighting AIDS). Notions of the 'gay community' rely on a shared understanding of an identity and culture. In this way, gay identity has been central in prevention efforts, many of which focus on establishing a safer sex or condom culture. This itself is dependent on the notion of a unitary gay identity. Indeed, HIV-prevention initiatives which have proved to be effective have been premised on just such gay community involvement (Kelly, St Lawrence and Diaz, 1991; Kelly *et al.*, 1992a). As such, community involvement is thought to be important because of the access it provides to informational resources (the gay press and safer sex information) and normative influences (descriptive and injunctive norms) and social support. Yet, despite the high profile of gay identity and gay community in both prevention initiatives and as theoretical constructs, the predictive validity of these constructs remains low. The majority of studies report non-significant associations between measures of sexual identity and changes in sexual behaviour (Hays, Kegeles and Coates, 1990; Doll *et al.*, 1991; Schmidt *et al.*, 1992).

Considering both the theoretical and the practical importance of sexual identity and gay community in gay men's sexual health, the low predictive validity of these constructs appears particularly surprising. However, these findings can partly be explained in terms of methodological problems. Because of the relative ease of sampling, much research on sexual health among gay men has been conducted with gay community samples drawn primarily from cohorts established in large cities with highly organized gay communities. As such, our existing knowledge-base about gay men's sexual health behaviour is predominantly drawn from urban, well-educated, white, middle-class, literate, employed, gay community-involved, self-identified gay men. These sampling issues are important as they question the applicability of the emerging knowledge-base about gay men's sexual health. Thus, despite the existence of a plurality of gay identities and gay communities, only one particular gay identity informs policy, research and prevention initiatives.

While the resulting information has been essential in assessing behavioural change in those men at most risk of HIV infection, its applicability to marginalized gay men and their communities remains questionable. Kelly *et al.* (1992b) point out that in the USA, 57 per cent of diagnosed AIDS cases have occurred outside San Francisco and the country's ten largest metropolitan areas. This bias is a particularly important issue in relation to the appropriateness of sexual health-promotional materials and interventions which were developed for, and targeted at, urban gay communities yet which are nevertheless employed outside these contexts. It is in contrast to unitary conceptions of gay identity, gay community and, indeed, sex, that this chapter attempts to describe the complexity of the links between sexual identities and sexual health.

Method

In-depth interviews were conducted with twenty men in the interviewee's own homes. All the men identified themselves as being gay and many of them reported engaging in sex with men who did not identify as gay. The participants were predominantly working-class, aged between 18 and 33 and all residents of Benton,[1] a small ex-mining town in South Yorkshire, England. All the participants were white. Only two had received higher education. The interviews were recorded on audiocassette and were transcribed verbatim. The names of all the men who took part in this study, and the people they have referred to, have been changed to ensure confidentiality. The transcripts were then analysed in terms of recurrent themes both within and across the interviews. Only data concerning sexual health and identity are examined here.

There are several qualitative methods that could be employed to look at themes and their relation to sexual behaviour. This chapter adopts a phenomenological approach, which takes people's accounts as indicative of their understandings of sexual behaviour. These understandings are seen to draw upon, and actively produce, the wider themes. This level of analysis retains the face validity of people's beliefs and attitudes. Furthermore, in exploring the connection between account, cognition and physical state, a useful framework is provided with which to combine data from other approaches such as social cognition (Smith, 1996).

The focus of this work is on men's understandings and not individual men *per se.* Although many men will share understandings, this does not apply to every single man. Moreover, any particular man may well have multiple and even contradictory understandings. The particular focus of analysis here is the understanding as opposed to the specific individual speakers. However, the analysis is presented through the use of individual extracts which retain some illustration of idiographic data, providing a supplementary level of insight. Particular extracts are chosen for each theme because they represent the most effective examples of the underlying themes.

The themes outlined below describe the salient identities which emerge within the interviews as having important effects on sexual decision-making and, indeed, sexual health decision-making. The themes illustrate the problematic nature of some implicit assumptions in sexual health research. As such they contrast the specific local experiences of gay men in Benton with the generalized claims of much quantitative sexual health theory.

Analysis

In Benton, sexual activity between men took place in two very distinct contexts. These contexts were described as 'on the scene' (in the only gay bar) and 'off the scene' (the latter mainly referred to cottaging).[2] Off the scene and within the cottage, men of apparently different sexual identities (both gay and straight) interacted in a way which was distinctly sexual as opposed to social. In contrast, on the scene, men's sexual activities could not clearly be separated from their social interactions. For men on the scene, the inseparable nature of gay men's social and sexual lives is best captured in the theme of reputation. This theme is presented first since the notion of reputation foregrounds the analysis and has consequences for the themes which are presented later. As such, the location of sexual activity is discussed as it relates to the dynamics of the encounters in which men of various sexual identities meet. Following this, some key features of the interactions between men of differing sexual identities are outlined in the theme of sex with straight men. Particular attention is paid to the notion of reciprocity. Finally, this notion and its implications about identity are discussed in the context of men who clearly identify with a gendered role in sexual activity. This is outlined in the theme of 'butch' and 'bitch'.

Reputation

Benton is a small community. It offers no choice of gay venues. In Benton there is a single pub which hosts two gay nights each week. This represented the focal point of the local gay community. Apart from this commercial venue, a sex sauna (which opened while the research was being conducted) and a local switchboard (which offers its services across the whole of South Yorkshire) represented the only accessible sites of the gay community. In this environment everyone seems to know everyone else. John gives some idea of where the local gay community can be found:

J. Erm, on market on a Friday, most of 'em are in market on a Friday morning.

P. Doing what?

J. Shopping! Some work on markets, I mean I know a few people that work on market, driving buses, erm, in cottages, most of 'em. Especially 'im from town hall, he's always in, I dun't know how he gets any work done, er, but you can guarantee no matter where you go, you allas bump into someone.

John describes a community in which it is possible to know and be known by most of the resident gay population. These circumstances facilitate a key notion that is very important in understanding sexual identities as they emerge within the interviews. This is reputation. People can become known, and indeed judged, as having certain reputations. These reputations often relate to the person's apparent willingness to have casual sex. Richard describes an encounter he had with a 'young guy' who was 'terribly, terribly camp'. He introduces the notion of reputation and outlines how this affected his sexual decision-making:

There was just something about him and somebody told me that he was a bit of a slag and you know, that he'd drop his pants for anybody and I thought 'Well, why not?' Terrible, I know, to use somebody like that.

Richard shows how the young guy's reputation invoked his identity as a slag. This was central in Richard's decision to have sex with him. Similarly, Nicholas describes how important reputation and its attendant identities are, this time in terms of who not to have sex with:

If you've been in a place a few times you hear, I mean there are certain people in Benton that you hear they're tarts, and I remember once being chatted up by a man and he was very nice looking, very nice indeed and I wasn't interested, I was going out with somebody and having heard more about him, I think he's not particularly choosy, put it that way, but he looked, you know, pretty nice, but he's not, it's just, you know, I wouldn't contemplate doing it with him if he wa' last person on earth.

It is interesting to note the force of reputation and the salience of its attendant identities (i.e. the 'slag', the 'tart', the 'slut'). Nicholas's sexual decision-making is clearly premised upon identity. In fact, Nicholas is willing to deny his own physical pleasure for fear of having sex with a tart. Within the interview when he was asked what he thought safer sex was, Nicholas replied it was 'not using condoms for a start'. For him sexual health decisions were made according to a partner's identity as a 'slag', a 'tart' or a 'slut'. Avoidance of these men was thought to be more of an effective risk-reduction strategy than condom use.

These extracts have highlighted how decisions relating to the choice of sexual partner are often made around the notions of identity and reputation. In the same way, the roles of reputation and identity are equally important in decisions relating to condom use. As Phil describes this:

P.   Why were you thinking about using condoms, then?

Ph. To be safe really, to be safe and to be clean, 'cos I mean he could have been with anybody. And I'd heard a few stories about him before and I heard a few after.

P.   What kind of stories had you heard about him?

Ph. He were Benton bike basically. Benton bike. Everybody had rode him basically. That's one of stories I'd heard and he'd got this and he'd got that and he'd got – I were really glad that I used some'at,[3] if I hadn't used owt I think I'd've ended up with some'at.

Previous quotes have shown how decisions relating to the choice of sexual partner are often related to reputation. Philip has described how the notion of reputation is also influential in people's decisions about condom use. Given the salience of reputation and the importance of the identities it highlights, it is not surprising that the fear of acquiring a negative reputation also emerges as important. As Richard says:

I frightened myself that I found it so easy to go off with people again and I just thought to myself if I don't calm myself down, I will end up doing this all the time and I won't find anybody because I will have been off with so many different people I'll just get a name for myself and I was terrified of that.

Richard hints at the apparent impossibility of finding a relationship because of the stigma of having a reputation as a 'slag'. In the next extract, Andrew

reiterates the perceived prohibition about engaging in casual sex. He also
outlines a distinct need to remain quiet about these activities:

A. Because it's not the done thing, you don't go around looking
    for sex in toilets.
P. Why?
A. Because it cheapens you, cheapens yourself, erm, basically it's
    not the done thing.
P. How do you mean it cheapens you?
A. Well, if you went around telling somebody that you went around
    looking for sex in toilets, you'd think, you'd just put yourself
    down saying it and the other persons thinking 'Well the dirty
    little slut!' you know, and you can see them thinking that, or
    'Does he have to resort to that sort of thing because he can't get
    a fella of his own?' sort of thing.

These understandings of reputation highlight the necessity of both guarding
and managing one's identity. They also highlight an important difference from
urban gay culture in what could be called 'sex-positivity'. Metropolitan gay
culture has a history of celebrating sex and sexual pleasure. A quick glance
through the popular gay press, particularly free newspapers in Britain such
as *Boyz*, assures one that this is still the case. In contrast to this, in small town
environments the notion of reputation invokes powerful prohibitions about
publicly acknowledging engaging in casual sex and outlines the importance
of a clearly sex-negative culture.

   In summary, this theme has outlined the importance of reputation in
terms of highlighting the lack of sex-positive culture. It has also described
the importance of the identity of the 'slag' in both sexual decision-making
(who to have sex with) and decisions relating to condom use. Although the
relation of reputation to sexual health promotion will be explored in the
discussion, it is also important in understanding the next two themes. First,
the notion of reputation helps to illuminate the dynamics of interactions in
public sex environments; and second, it is important in addressing gay men's
accounts of sex between men of differing sexual identities.

The Location of Sex and Identity

The previous theme outlined a general prohibition on casual sex for gay
men who frequented the gay scene in Benton. The risk of being identified
as a 'slag' or a 'slut' minimizes willingness to publicly acknowledge engaging
in casual sex. Much of the casual sex in Benton took place off the scene and
in cottages. The cottage represents a particular social environment in which

identity remains ambiguous. Sexual motivation is cloaked under the guise of toilet use. Men referred to the diversity of what they called 'trade', reflecting the variety of men who go cottaging. Trade is a wide-reaching catch-all term that reflects not only gay identified men such as those who took part in this study, but a host of other identified men who could all be classified under the ubiquitous 'men who have sex with men' (MSM). Within the interviews these MSM's were named as 'married gay men', 'cottage queens', 'chickens', 'bisexuals', 'old queens' and 'straight men'. As this theme shows, the cottage provides a forum in which identities are suspended and sexual motivation is masked. Gay men can avoid the complications of casual sex on the scene, straight men can engage in sex with other men without risking their straight identities, and all men can avoid the explicit articulation of sexual identities altogether. In the cottage, sexual partners who do not go out on the gay scene can be found without risking one's reputation. This stands in contrast to the public scrutiny of their sex life on the gay scene and the inevitability of talking and socializing with partners (particularly if partners return to the home and the bed). In these domestic situations, conversation is unavoidable and anonymity is lost. Daniel was asked if there were any differences between cottaging and sex in the home, he replied of the former:

> Yeah, it's more disposable. Well, it is disposable sex, that's the whole thing about it. It's quick, cheap and cheerful. You don't have any of the problems of taking someone back and to talk to them and what have you.

Dan's description of sex centres around its simplicity and the very lack of inter-personal interaction. He can have sex with someone and keep it as 'disposable sex'. By doing this he can avoid, in his words, the problem of talking to some-one. Through describing it as disposable, Dan captures a sense of it as having a one-off (or throw away) function. If we consider the social costs for gay men engaging in casual sex under the judgmental eye of the tightly knit local gay community, we can see how the cottage represents a unique opportunity to engage in casual sex. Within a cottage, the constant fear of interruption by the police or other toilet users ensures a speedy interaction, minimal conversation, maximum anonymity and necessitates very limited personal involvement. With respect to these constraints, the interviews describe a struggle to maintain the appearance of toilet use while simultaneously engaging in sex. John succinctly describes how this affects sexual decision-making:

> You've always got to be on your guard, so you can't relax, I mean you can't turn around when somebody's got his dick up your arse and say 'I'm just having a pee' (laughs).

John describes how, at a urinal, contextual constraints limit the possible re-pertoire of sexual acts. However, not all of the encounters initiated within the cottage led to sex within the cottage. Men talked of leaving to go to other quieter cottages, cars or partner's homes. This negotiation of further location was often conducted in the form of notes passed under walls or between toilet cubicles. Yet, if sex partners remain within the cottage, behaviour and sexual decisions are limited by the dynamics of that specific location. These demand that men engaging in sexual activity are not immediately identifiable as such. Instead, they must appear as *bona fide* toilet users. If men do not wish to stand at the urinal then there is scope for sex in toilet cubicles. This location facilitates a different set of behavioural rules including a longer time period for sexual activity. Neil describes how this affects sexual decision-making:

> Whereas a cubicle, one, you can spend at least ten minutes sat down there and anybody comes into there and says 'What's he doing?' It's obvious you're having a dump, so there's a lot more excuse to be there. Even though you're not – you're really having a peep show.

Neil describes the importance of remaining identifiable as a toilet user as opposed to a cottager. He describes the deliberate management of his appearance.

Similarly, Peter describes why he chose to use glory holes[4] in cubicles. His reasons for having sex in this context relate not only to the pressures of apparent toilet use but also to the apparent meaning of this sexual activity:

> Then I found toilets with holes in, with bits taken out of partitions and that. That was ... I found that a lot better 'cos I could sit and ... I didn't have to look at them, talking to them and I never see them again. I mean you can say that the eye-to-eye contact wasn't there and I wasn't open for people to talk to me and that is still ... now, I don't like people to talk to me. I don't mind doing it with ugly guys but if I'm cruising somebody up I don't like them to talk to me during any part of cruising.

Peter highlights a preference for an interaction that remains non-verbal, purely physical and totally anonymous. Through using the glory hole, Peter's partners could quite literally be anybody. These men had no face, no whole body and no identity. As Peter noted he will never see them again; they too are completely disposable.

In summary, this theme has described how sexual decisions (about the choice of sexual acts) are often constrained by the situational dynamics of the location of sexual activity. These dynamics also provide a unique opportunity for gay men to engage in sex with others and avoid social interaction. By choosing to have casual sex in these locations, gay men minimize the risk to their reputations through the particular dynamics of the cottage (e.g. the appearance of toilet use). This ensures an ambiguity which masks their sexual activities and hides other non-gay-identified men's sexual motivation. Furthermore, by choosing to have sex in a cottage, men are less likely to meet their contemporaries from the scene. They are also more likely to meet men who do not go out in the gay social world – or as the next theme describes them, straight and bisexual men.

Sex with Straight Men

The minimal interactions which locations like the cottage provide, not only offer gay men the opportunity to engage in casual sex, but also offer men who do not identify as gay the opportunity to engage in sex with other men while avoiding the stigma of a gay identity. Within the interviews, such activity was often described, not as sex, but as 'relief'. The term 'relief' is used as a description of other people's assumed motivation to have sex. In using relief as a motivation for activities which could be construed as sexual, much of the contradiction in popular understandings of sexual identity can be accommodated. Relief captures a sense of a purely somatic phenomenon, of an almost involuntary need. By minimizing the significance of the activity, a coherent sexual identity remains possible despite the practice of seemingly contradictory sexual behaviour. Dan shows how these identities emerge within these, often non-verbal, sexual encounters:

> That's the big thing, a lot of sort of casual sex where some people don't like snogging and they don't snog. It's like a lot of straight people use them (cottages) and it's a way of distancing, distancing yourself from it. Doing it with your body but not with your mind.

As Dan's account suggests, the practice and avoidance of some specific acts in specific contexts (i.e. 'snogging' in a cottage) can be used to maintain an apparent sexual identity – a straight identity – while simultaneously engaging in contradictory behaviour. Simon expands on this:

> It's usually, I always find it's usually been like, bisexual men and I always think it's like 'Oh, we haven't kissed you, so we're not doing anything like,' they've just like done everything else to you but like, 'we haven't kissed you, so we're not gay or we're not bisexual, we haven't kissed you', I just don't understand it.

Again, it is clear that sexual decisions (the choice of sexual acts) have been made around the dictates of sexual identities. This understanding of kissing is so strong that both Daniel and Simon have described how plausible sexual identities might be maintained despite an apparent contradiction in sexual behaviour. The nature of some interactions between gay and apparently straight men draws attention to the notion of reciprocity. Between men, the possibility of perfect reciprocity, and variations from it, also provide a prime site for the articulation of specific meanings and identities. As Rob explains:

> R. When we are talking about cottaging we like split it in half because some people don't go out on the scene, some people are bisexual or married or just want to go in for a bit of relief, you know.
> P. So can you tell the difference between these types of people?
> R. Yeah, you can really, by what they do, because usually they don't . . . for some, I don't even know if they're bisexual because some don't even touch you, some just want a blow job or a wank and that's it, they don't even think about touching you.

Rob illustrates an apparent division of sexual motivation. The straight man was seeking 'relief' and the gay man wanted 'sex'. The central point Rob makes is the link between reciprocity and sexual identity. Through not reciprocating in some activities, men reportedly displayed a distinct lack of interest in their partners, both as people and even as sex objects. The decisions about the choice of sexual acts were constrained by the links between certain acts and identity.

Simon described the differences between sex with gay men and sex with straight or bisexual men:

> A gay man, if he's enjoyed himself, what you've done with him, will reciprocate and make sure you've enjoyed what's gone on. A straight or bi man will take, take, take. He's not interested in what you've had out of it, or if you've enjoyed it. He's just had what he wants and that's all that matters. That all comes from how it's been through the centuries. You know women, you know kitchen women,[5] they look at gay men or an affair as the same sort of thing. You're there for their use and there's no interest that you've enjoyed it, it's roll over and do it, 'cos I want. Two gay men together, I think we have a better understanding and a softer approach and whatever else and that's why you're more caring and making sure the other person's enjoying it as well, I mean not everybody but generally.

Simon's description highlights the distinction between sex that is about bodies and sex that is also about the people concerned. He clearly illustrates the mapping of sexual identities across this divide. For Simon, straight men are concerned only with their own physical needs, while he believes gay men relate to each other primarily as people (with sexual needs) but not solely as sex objects.

What emerges from these extracts is an understanding of the complex relationship between sexual identity and context. In situations such as the cottage where there is no verbal interaction, sexual identities must always be supposed. There is little scope for conversation and apparent identities emerge from a detailed language of reciprocity and assumed motivation in genital activity (relief versus sex). By invoking a partner's straight sexual identity and his lack of interest in a gay man as a person, it is clear that culpability about the casual nature of the sexual activity remains clearly with the straight man. In terms of the effects of sexual identity on sexual decision-making, it appears that particular sexual acts were avoided solely because of their association with particular sexual identities. This issue relates to the next theme which addresses particular links between the notion of reciprocity, the choice of sexual acts and the emergence of further identities.

'Butch' and 'Bitch'

The previous extracts outlined the importance of ideas of reciprocity in differentiating between emergent sexual identities such as gay and straight. Unlike sex between a man and a woman, there is the possibility of absolute reciprocity in sex between men since each body is anatomically similar. As the last theme described, asymmetry in sexual behaviour can articulate quite specific identities. The theme of 'butch' and 'bitch' identities further explores the notion of reciprocity and investigates some of those meanings relating to asymmetrical penetrative sex between men.

While many men saw receptive anal sex as being a reciprocal activity like any other which both partners could enjoy, many of the men also expressed a distinct understanding of asymmetry in penetrative sex. Philip introduces the key concepts here: 'I wanted to be fucked basically. To see what it were like, to see whether I did like it, to make me decision whether I were going to be bitch or butch.' He outlines the distinction between 'butch' or 'bitch' which stems from a preference for being either insertive or receptive in anal intercourse. Philip presents it as a dichotomous decision which will have consequences for him as a person. It directly relates to his identification with a preference for being receptive or insertive. By being penetrated and receiving a partner's penis into one's body and not reciprocating (fucking one's partner) a gendered identity seems to emerge. This gendered identity relates the receptive body to what is described by the men who took part in this study as a 'female' identity. As Nicholas describes it:

N.   I think, erm, I don't know, I feel a bit silly saying this, but, I feel almost like a girl, you know what I mean, like I think, you take sort of like a man sort of thing and a woman. I mean Kev used to call me his girlfriend or his niece or some'at like that, although it weren't a particularly power sort of thing it wa'

> more of a sex gender sort of thing, and he used to say that and
> as daft as sounds, almost, you know, you used to think, well yeah,
> alright sort of thing.
>
> P.   What, it turned you on him saying that?
>
> N.   Yeah, it did actually, I've got to say, not turn me on as much, but
> you know, I liked it, yeah, it did I've got to say . . . I think a lot
> of people, you know tend to see younger people, or definitely
> younger people who are passive, I mean they say 'she' when they're
> talking about things like that, you'll have noticed that yourself.

Nicholas describes how gender is appropriated from an understanding of
reciprocity in penetrative sex. Richard describes how he felt this was relevant
for his relationship in general:

> I always used to think that if you were the one doing the fucking, you
> were the dominant one, like the male and the submissive partner was
> like the weakest one and so like you were the boss all the time, you
> know what I mean.

Richard reiterates the gendered aspect of a lack of reciprocity in anal sex.
Through equating being insertive with a male identity and being receptive
with a female identity, a simple understanding of being gay in terms of a
single homosexuality becomes inadequate. Whereas being gay is often understood to relate to the involvement of the respective male identities and male
bodies in sexual acts, being either butch or bitch complicates this simple
understanding. Sex between two men can be understood as: sex between
'male' and 'female' identities; sex between two 'female' identities; or sex
between two male identities. This understanding is premised on the denial of
anatomical and somatic understandings of sex and instead is centred around
the gendered identity of self and other. Furthermore, a 'heterosexual' coupling
is the desired outcome. Sexual decisions are again constrained by identity: in
this case the choice of sexual acts must necessarily be penetrative and necessarily asymmetrical. In other words, decisions around anal penetration are
based around 'bitch' and 'butch' identities. As Philip says of his friend Pete:

> It's like me friend, Pete, he's strictly bitch and if you said to 'im 'Did
> you have a shag last night?', 'Well, yeah, but I were shagged,' 'Oh,
> did you shag him?', 'Oh, God! Don't make me feel sick, if I'm gunna
> shag him I might as well go with a woman.'

Philip outlines how anatomical sex can be understood as unimportant. Instead,
the gendered identity stemming from a lack of reciprocity in penetrative
sex is seen as central. Sexual decision-making is again constrained by identity. It can be seen that if anatomical sex is not requisite for sexual activity
or relationships, then one must determine a potential partner's gender as

the opposite to one's own. Thus, a 'bitch' man would want a 'butch' man as a partner and vice versa, as Rob says: 'A camp queen isn't going to go with another camp queen, is it?'

It thus becomes essential to find out someone's gendered identity. Decisions around sex are made around notions of these identities. Philip describes how difficult this process can be:

> Ph. Like the young chap that you met when you came in, well, I was so determined that he was strictly butch but when I got him into bed and I thought 'Oh, God, he's got to be butch, he's got to be butch' and he turned out bitch and it were just like 'I can't do with this, I can't do with this, the only thing we're gunna be able to do is just rub fannies together' and that's all it wa'.
>
> P. So how did you determine that he was bitch and not butch?
>
> Ph. Well, I sat on top of him and he kept shoving away and I'm thinking 'this is not right', well and he hadn't even got an 'ardon,[6] and I thought a lot of strictly bitch people dun't even get an 'ardon 'cos it dun't even bother 'em and there were just no 'ardon at all and I'm thinking to me sen[7] 'there's some'at wrong 'ere.'

Philip describes his difficulty in correctly assessing the gendered identity of his partner. In keeping with the bitch identity, it is interesting to note the use of terms usually used to describe female genitalia (fannies) to describe their penises. Philip also shows how the gendered sex of the body is played down through noting the lack of attention given to the penis and ejaculation that a bitch shows through a distinct focus upon the anus and the receptive role.

In summary, the singular notion of gay identity in explaining sexual decisions for gay men in Benton seems limited. A unitary conception of gay identity fails to capture the salience of gendered identities such as bitch and butch. Decisions about penetrative sexual activity are necessarily constrained by these identities. These identities highlight normative expectations of penetrative sex and also draw attention to the importance of receptive or insertive roles in penetrative sex and highlight what appears to be an apparent sex-role rigidity. The identities of butch and bitch were a regular feature of the social world of gay men in Benton and familiar to all the men who took part in this study.

Discussion

Dowsett, Davis and Connell (1992, p. 316) address the paucity of research about the impact of class on sexual identity, sexual health and HIV-prevention.

They note that 'less advantaged men live less segregated from heterosexual social life compared with more affluent gay men, and also that they had less access to educational and informational resources about HIV/AIDS'. They highlight the necessity of recognizing both the similarities and the differences between affluent gay men who participate in an emergent international gay culture, and the experiences of other men and communities that are excluded and marginalized from that gay culture. The present study can be understood as outlining some of these differences and similarities in the context of Benton.

The idea of reputation highlighted the importance of identities such as the 'slag', in terms of sexual health decision-making (both who to have sex with and condom use). Research among heterosexuals has highlighted similar understandings (Kitzinger, 1993; Waldby, Kippax and Crawford, 1993). The latter utilize the notion of a '*cordon sanitaire*', this is a way of structuring the chaos of potentially infectious social and sexual worlds. It divides the clean from the unclean and seeks to map out a margin of safety, one that outlines apparent strategies for sexual health. In this way, potential or actual sexual partners are differentiated in terms of their clean/unclean status and decisions relating to condom use are made accordingly.

Precisely the same ideas can be seen in some of the men's statements reported here. Reputation is dependent on a specific social context wherein people repeatedly meet each other and become identifiable to each other. This makes it possible for potential partners to be identifiable as either clean or unclean. Here, the salience of identities such as the 'slag' highlight the need for sexual health promotion to address beliefs which posit risk in terms of particular people and not particular sexual acts. The role of reputation, like that of 'negotiated safety' (Kippax *et al.*, 1993) is an example, albeit an ineffective one, of the complexity and sophistication of gay men's HIV risk-reduction strategies. These stand in contrast to sexual health promotion's unitary and often simplistic response to the threat of HIV infection.

In Benton, there is a distinct lack of the sex-positive values associated with metropolitan gay culture. This is a particularly important issue in relation to the transfer of sexual health-promotion materials from large urban, sex-positive gay communities to communities like Benton. The importance of reputation also highlights the relative ease of reaching most of the gay community. The tightness of social networks lends itself to peer-education strategies, for example, those based around ideas of diffusion of innovation (Rogers, 1983).

The second theme focused on the location of sexual activity. It described how sexual decisions (concerning the choice of sexual acts) were often constrained by the situational dynamics of the location of sexual activity. These dynamics mask sexual motivation and obscure identities. The appearance of toilet use in the cottage provided gay men with the opportunity to engage in casual sex with other men. The cottage also represented the chance for men without gay identities to engage in sex with other men, without risking their straight identities. With regard to sexual decision-making, it could be argued that many decisions relating to choice of sexual acts are based around the dynamics of the location and are unaffected by notions of HIV risk. Within the cottage, sex was unlikely to be penetrative and the meaning of certain acts such as kissing also influenced sexual decision-making. Kissing had connotations of interpersonal involvement and was avoided precisely because of these meanings. The literature about sexual location and sexual activity is also sparse. Laud Humphrey's (1970) famous study *Tearoom Trade* has been supplemented by more recent behavioural studies such as Church *et al.* (1993) and Bennett, Chapman and Bray (1989).

With regards to sexual health promotion for men who remain within the cottage, verbal interaction is severely constrained. There is little scope for the dissemination of HIV-prevention messages. However, the dynamics of sex in this location ensure that the activity is relatively safe (either oral sex or masturbation). Yet when men leave the cottage to engage in sex (which may be penetrative), there is scope for HIV-preventive education as conversation becomes inevitable. In these situations, as this chapter has indicated, gay men mix sexually with 'hard to reach' men. However, the extent to which these interactions provide a viable forum for the transfer of a safer sex culture remains an open question.

The theme of straight identities focused on the complex interrelationship between sexual identity and context. Building on issues surrounding the location of sexual activity, this theme examined sexual identities in context. In the cottage, conversation is effectively outlawed and imputed sexual identities emerge from a language of reciprocity and assumed motivation within sexual activity. Decisions relating to sexual activity are constrained both by location and the articulation of these identities, through, for example, not kissing and not reciprocating in masturbation and oral sex. The literature about sex between men without gay identities is also sparse. Earl (1990, p. 256) briefly outlines some aspects of such encounters and concludes that 'this is a difficult population to reach as their forms of denial are selective, clearly self-serving, and insulated by their ties to the heterosexual culture'. Similarly, Bennett, Chapman and Bray (1989), Doll *et al.* (1992) and Siebt, McAllister and Freeman (1991) all report data addressing levels of risk behaviour among non-gay-identified men but do not examine the social context of such activity.

The notion of reciprocity is further developed in discussing the theme of butch and bitch identities. These identities again constrain sexual decision-making by ensuring that sexual activity must be penetrative and that the receptive or insertive roles are identity-specific. The literature about cross-cultural studies of homosexuality is insightful here (Carrier, 1971, 1976; Lancaster, 1988; Parker, 1989). For example, Parker notes that in Brazil there is a particular cultural emphasis on gender roles as opposed to sexual practices. He notes that 'the symbolic structure of male/female interactions seems to function in many ways as a kind of model for the organisation of same sex interactions in Brazilian culture. Within the terms of this model, what is centrally important is perhaps less the shared biological gender of the participants than the social roles they play out' (Parker, 1989, p. 273). In Benton, the same prioritization of social roles is visible with the disavowal of biological gender and the appropriation of gendered identities. These findings highlight the danger of sexual health promotion which seeks to promote non-penetrative sex, as this would clearly be culturally inappropriate.

The salience of factors other than sensate pleasure and disease avoidance are clearly important in both sexual decision-making and as influencing condom use. They reflect the importance of examining sexual behaviour beyond the sexual health paradigm and thus beyond traditional models of health psychology. Variables drawn from health psychological models remain poor at predicting sexual behaviour change (Flowers *et al.*, 1996). Rhodes (1995, p. 128) describes such theories as 'single rationality theories of risk' wherein the individual always seeks to maximize their health. Decisions about the choice of sexual acts are conceived of as cost-and-benefit analyses, in which an individual's disease-prevention beliefs are weighed against an individual's beliefs about sexual pleasure (loss of sensation). These models are epidemiologically driven and focus on a somatic understanding of sex. They see the individual's sexual decision-making as being a rational health-related choice. Clearly there is a growing body of work which highlights the inadequacy of this understanding and highlights the plethora of other motivations or 'rationalities'. It is the juxtaposition of these motivations in relation to a unitary conceptualization of sexual activity that has become problematic in sexual health research. There are parallels with the literature about heterosexuals (Hollway, 1984; Holland, Ramazanoglu and Scott, 1990; Wight, 1993).

Bloor (1995) and Rhodes (1995) highlight the utility of situated rationality theories of risk which accommodate a plurality of other possible rationalities. In this way, cost-and-benefit analyses can include the social costs of arrest within cottaging weighed against the benefits of engaging in anal sex, or the benefits of communicating intimacy and trust with a lover as compared to HIV risk from unprotected anal intercourse (Flowers *et al.*, 1997). In this way, situated rationality theories move beyond a unitary somatic understanding of sex and instead suggest sex can be seen as a repertoire of physical activities which potentially have a plethora of different meanings. These meanings inform both sexual decisions and sexual health decisions. Thus, this understanding explores sexual behaviour outside a purely 'health' perspective and illustrates the limitations of understanding sexual behaviour solely from this perspective. Models of sexual decision-making should begin with some contextualizing of the sex in terms of its motivation – whether it be concerned with the dynamics of a relationship, identity (Ingham, Woodcock and Stenner, 1992), economic influences (Zalduondo and Bernard, 1995) or of power (Holland, Ramazanoglu and Scott, 1990; Bloor *et al.*, 1992) or solely of sexual pleasure.

In conclusion, the utility of unitary understandings of gay identity, sex and even risk is limited. Theories of sexual health must accommodate the many diverse understandings of sex in order to be effective in informing sexual health-promotion practice. In turn, sexual health-promotion practice must address sexual behaviour beyond the somatic guise of condom provision and move towards responding to risk as it is experienced by gay men themselves.

Notes

1   'Benton' is a pseudonym.
2   Cottaging refers to sexual activity occurring within public toilets.
3   'Something'.
4   A glory hole is a hole between toilet cubicles, or between a toilet cubicle and the main body of a public toilet. It is used for sex, the penis being put through the hole thus allowing certain sexual activities to occur.
5   This is an abbreviated form of the proverb 'women who are tied to the kitchen sink'.
6   'Hard on' or erection.
7   'Myself'.

References

BENNET, G., CHAPMAN, S. and BRAY, F. (1989) 'Sexual practices and "Beats": AIDS-related sexual practices in a sample of homosexual and bisexual men in the western area of Sydney', *The Medical Journal of Australia*, **151**, pp. 309–14.

BLOOR, M.J. (1995) 'A user's guide to contrasting theories of HIV-related risk behaviour', in J. GABE (Ed.) *Health Medicine and Risk: The Need for a Sociological Approach*, Oxford: Blackwell.

BLOOR, M.J., McKEGANEY, N.P., FINLAY, A. and BARNARD, M.A. (1992) 'The inappropriateness of psycho-social models of risk behaviour for understanding HIV-related risk practices among Glasgow male prostitutes', *AIDS Care*, **4**, pp. 131–7.

BOLTON, R. (1992) 'Mapping *terra incognita*: sex research for AIDS prevention – an urgent agenda for the 1990s', in G. HERDT and S. LINDENBAUM (Eds) *In the Time of AIDS*, California: Newbury Park.

BOULTON, M., McLEAN, J., FITZPATRICK, R. and HART, G. (1995) 'Gay men's accounts of unsafe sex', *AIDS Care*, **7**, pp. 619–30.

CALLEN (1983) *How to have sex in an epidemic*, New York: News from the Front Publications.

CARRIER, J.M. (1971) 'Sex role preference as an explanatory variable in homosexual behaviour', *Archives of Sexual Behaviour*, **6**, pp. 53–65.

CARRIER, J.M. (1976) 'Cultural factors affecting urban Mexican male homosexual behaviour', *Archives of Sexual Behaviour,* **5**, pp. 103–24.

CATANIA, J.A., GIBSON, D.R., CHITWOOD, D.D. and COATES T.J. (1990) 'Methodological problems in AIDS behavioural research: influences on measurement error and participation bias in studies of sexual behaviour', *Psychological Bulletin,* **108**, pp. 339–62.

CHURCH, J., GREEN, J., VEARNALS, S. and KEOGH, P. (1993) 'Investigation of motivational and behavioural factors influencing men who have sex with other men in public toilets (cottaging)', *AIDS Care,* **5**, pp. 337–46.

DOLL, L.S., PETERSON, L.R., WHITE, C.R., JOHNSON, E.S. and WARD, J.W. and the blood-donor study group (1992) 'Homosexually and non-homosexually identified men: a behavioural comparison', *Journal of Sex Research,* **29**, pp. 1–14.

DOLL, L.S., BYERS, R.H., BOLAN, G., DOUGLAS, J.M., MOSS P.M., WELLER, P.D., JOY, D. *et al.* (1991) 'Homosexual men who engage in high-risk sexual behaviour: a multicenter comparison', *Sexually Transmitted Diseases,* **18**, pp. 170–5.

DOWSETT, G.W., DAVIS, M.D. and CONNELL, R.W. (1992) 'Working-class homosexuality and HIV/AIDS prevention: some recent research from Sydney, Australia', *Psychology and Health,* **6**, pp. 313–24.

EARL, W.L. (1990) 'Married men and same sex activity: a field study of HIV risk among men who do not identify as gay or bisexual', *Journal of Sex and Marital Therapy,* **16**, pp. 251–7.

FLOWERS, P., SHEERAN, P., BEAIL, N. and SMITH, J.A. (1996) 'The role of psychosocial factors in HIV risk-reduction among gay and bisexual men: a quantitative review', *Psychology and Health* (in press).

FLOWERS, P., SMITH, J.A., SHEERAN, P. and BEAIL, N. (1997) 'Health and Romance: Understanding unprotected sex in relationships between gay men', *British Journal of Health Psychology* (in press).

GLASER, B. and STRAUSS, A. (1967) *The Discovery of Grounded Theory,* Chicago: Aldine.

HAYS, R.B., KEGELES, S.M. and COATES, T.J. (1990) 'High HIV risk-taking among young gay men', *AIDS,* **4**, pp. 901–7.

HART, G. and BOULTON, M. (1995) 'Sexual behaviour in gay men: towards a sociology of risk', in P. AGGLETON, P. DAVIES and G. HART (Eds) *AIDS: Safety, Sexuality and Risk,* London: Taylor & Francis.

HOLLAND, J., RAMAZANOGLU, C. and SCOTT, S. (1990) 'Managing risk and experiencing danger: tensions between government AIDS health education policy and young women's sexuality', *Gender and Education,* **2**, pp. 125–9.

HOLLAND, J., RAMAZANOGLU, C., SCOTT, S., SHARPE, S. and THOMSON, R. (1991) 'Between embarrassment and trust: young women and the diversity of condom use', in P. AGGLETON, G. HART and P. DAVIES (Eds) *AIDS: Responses, Interventions and Care,* London: Falmer Press.

HOLLWAY, W. (1984) 'Gender difference and the production of subjectivity', in J. HENRIQUES, W. HOLLWAY, C. URWIN, C. VENN, and V. WALKERDINE (Eds) *Changing the Subject: Psychology, Social Regulation and Subjectivity,* London: Methuen.

HUMPHREYS, L. (1970) *Tearoom Trade,* Chicago: Aldine.

INGHAM, R., WOODCOCK, A. and STENNER, K. (1992) 'The limitations of rational decision-making models as applied to young people's sexual behaviour', in P. AGGLETON, P. DAVIES and G. HART (Eds) *AIDS: Rights, Risk and Reason*, London: Falmer Press.

KELLY, J.A., ST LAWRENCE, J.S. and DIAZ, Y.E. (1991) 'HIV risk behaviour reduction following intervention with key opinion leaders of a population: an experimental community level analysis', *American Journal of Public Health*, **81**, pp. 168–71.

KELLY, J.A., ST LAWRENCE, J.S., STEVENSON, L.Y., HAUTH, A.C., KALICHMAN, S.C., DIAZ, Y.E., BRASFIELD, T.L. *et al.* (1992a) 'Community AIDS/HIV risk reduction: the effects of endorsements by popular people in three cities', *American Journal of Public Health*, **82**, pp. 1483–9.

KELLY, J.A., MURPHY, D., ROFFMAN, R.A., SOLOMAN, L.J., WINETT, R.A., STEVENSON, L.Y., KOOB, J.J. *et al.* (1992b) 'Acquired immunodeficiency syndrome/human immunodeficiency virus risk behaviour among gay men in small cities: findings from a 16-city national sample', *Archives of Internal Medicine*, **152**, pp. 2293–7.

KING, E. (1993) *Safety in Numbers*, London: Cassell.

KIPPAX, S., CRAWFORD, J., DAVIS, M., RODDEN P. and DOWSETT, G. (1993) 'Sustaining safe sex: a longitudinal study of a sample of homosexual men', *AIDS*, **7**, pp. 257–63.

KITZINGER, J. (1993) 'Safer sex and dangerous reputations: contradictions for young women negotiating condom use', MRC Medical Sociology Unit, Working Paper No. 47.

LANCASTER, R.N. (1988) 'Subject honour and object shame: the construction of male homosexuality and stigma in nicaragua', *Ethnology*, **27**, pp. 111–25.

MURRAY, S.O. (1992) 'The 'underdevelopment' of modern gay homosexuality in Meso–America', in K. PLUMMER (Ed.) *Modern Homosexualities: Fragments of a Gay and Lesbian Experience*, London: Routledge.

PARKER, R. (1989) 'Youth, identity, and homosexuality: the changing shape of sexual life in contemporary Brazil', *Journal of Homosexuality*, **17**, pp. 269–89.

PRIEUR, A. (1990) 'Gay men: reasons for continued practice of unsafe sex', *AIDS Education and Prevention*, **2**, pp. 110–17.

RHODES, T. (1995) 'Theorizing and researching "risk": notes on the social relations of risk in heroin users "lifestyles"', in P. AGGLETON, P. DAVIES and G. HART (Eds) *AIDS: Safety, Sexuality and Risk*, London: Taylor & Francis.

ROGERS, E.M. (1983) *Diffusion of Innovations*. New York: Free Press.

SCHMIDT, K.W., FOUCHARD, J.R., KRASNIK, A., ZOFFMANN, H., JACOBSEN H.L. and KREINER, S. (1992) 'Sexual behaviour related to psychosocial factors in a population of Danish homosexual and bisexual men', *Social Science and Medicine*, **34**, pp. 1119–27.

SHILTS, R. (1987) *And the Band Played On: People, Politics and the AIDS Crisis*, Harmondsworth: Penguin Books.

SIEBT, A.C., McALLISTER, A.L. and FREEMAN, A.C. (1991) 'Condom use and sexual identity among men who have sex with men – Dallas', *Morbidity and Mortality Weekly Reports*, **42**, pp. 12–13.

SMITH, J.A. (1996) 'Beyond the divide between cognition and discourse: using interpretative phenomenological analysis in health psychology', *Psychology and Health*, 11, pp. 261–71.

SPEARS, R., ABRAHAM, S.C.S., ABRAMS, D. and SHEERAN, P. (1992) 'Framing in terms of "high-risk" groups versus "risky practices" and prognoses of HIV infection', *European Journal of Social Psychology*, 22, pp. 195–201.

WALDBY, C., KIPPAX, S. and CRAWFORD, J. (1993) '*Cordon sanitaire*: "Clean" and "unclean" women in the AIDS discourse of young heterosexual men', in P. AGGLETON, P. DAVIES and G. HART (Eds) *AIDS: Facing the Second Decade*, London, Taylor & Francis.

WIGHT, D. (1993) 'Assimilating "safer sex": young heterosexual men's understanding of "safer sex"', paper presented at the seventh conference on Social Aspects of AIDS, South Bank University, London.

ZALDUONDO, B. and BERNARD, J.M. (1995) 'Meanings and consequences of sexual-economic exchange: gender, poverty and sexual risk behaviour in urban Haiti', in R. PARKER and J.H. GAGNON (Eds) *Conceiving Sexuality: Approaches to Sex Research in a Post-modern World*, London: Routledge.

Chapter 13

State-sponsored Gayness: Ghettoization as a Response to HIV/AIDS

Gary Smith and Michael Bartos

In the contemporary world, becoming gay requires becoming other. For much of this century gayness has been understood in terms of a perversion or deviation from a (hetero)sexual object choice, whose pathology was to be understood in terms of arrested or malformed development. Gay Liberation intended to change such notions, but even in these liberal times, being a gay man or a lesbian still requires a deliberate differentiation from a background of presumptive heterosexuality.

The ghettoization of gayness is a process of social and geographic consolidation, the construction of homosexual desire and the suppression of that desire in dominant culture. Gay liberationists saw coming out as a political response on the part of the self-identified gay person to their social oppression (Weeks, 1977; Cain, 1991). Coming out was largely conceptualized as a collective rather than an individual response to heterosexism, laying the groundwork for the creation of a gay community.

By the mid- to late-1970s, this community-building work was seen to have a spatialized dimension, with the creation of visibly gay (and sometimes lesbian) districts in a number of cities. The development of spatially located homosexual subcultures has been traced back much earlier, to the formation of large urban centres, such as London, in the seventeenth century (Bray, 1982). The commercialized urban gay centres of contemporary Western society are the most recent permutation in the history of homosexual subcultural formation, adding a politics of visibility and liberation to the long-standing existence of specific places for the pursuit of pleasure. While the notion of ghetto has been criticized by some cultural geographers as too simplistic a reduction of gay identity to gay places (Davis, 1995), in certain cities, of which Sydney is one, there remains a palpable concatenation of gay geographies, identities, institutions and an economy that deserves to retain the name *ghetto*.

This chapter considers some of the most recent developments in the contemporary processes of coming to a gay identity and practice and, in particular, the way in which the formation of gay identity has fallen into the domain of public health in those countries where sex between men is a major route of HIV transmission. In the past fifteen years, coming out has become institutionalized as part of the gay community's response to AIDS. Herdt contends that the era of AIDS constitutes a major historical and cultural shift for the emergence of gay and lesbian identities, and that for the first time 'an institutionalised process of initiating and socialising [gay and lesbian] youths has emerged' (Herdt, 1992, p. 34). AIDS created an urgent need to educate homosexual men (in particular) about how to avoid becoming infected with HIV, or for those who were already infected, to cope with the social and health issues the disease posed. In the name of public health, coming out has been institutionally facilitated through strategies of gay community development and community attachments (Dowsett, 1990a). In Australia, the key community attachment strategy has been peer education, particularly in relation to youth (Feachem, 1995). The basic process of youth peer education is to facilitate young gay men's transition into gay culture and to impart and consolidate norms of safe sex that are integral to that culture.

All gay men and lesbians have a story to tell about the tension between homosexuality and heterosexuality, a tension which is typically resolved through the development of a homosexual identity or consciousness. For many, the means of resolving the tension is to *come out* and adopt a gay or lesbian identity.[1] This chapter draws on 23 semi-structured in-depth interviews with young gay men aged between 17 and 25 who attended HIV peer education youth groups in three major urban areas of New South Wales, Australia.[2] Ten of the men were followed up after a one-year period. The interviews lasted from one to two hours and covered a range of themes including sexual practice, the disclosure of homosexuality, sexual identity, involvement in gay community, work and family history.

Given these men were recruited through youth groups, their experiences illuminate the intersection between coming out and government-funded community-development projects. They provide an exemplary site to research young men's development of a gay identity within state-funded organizations. Most of the men had recently begun to disclose their homosexuality to other people and it was generally the case that social and familial networks discouraged or disapproved of the men's homosexuality. Attending the youth groups was often the first step these men took to establish a homosexual network.

The interview data was analysed in terms of the pathways through which the young men entered into sexual and social homosexual networks. The information was then related to the logic of HIV public health policy within Australia.

Entry into Gay Community

The model of peer education and gay community development which emerged as an institutional response to AIDS has harnessed coming out to serve public health needs. Starting with experience which may be tentative or confusing, it aims to mesh homosexual desire and social identity into a singular, comfortable gay identity. The goal is to achieve an integrated personality, and coming out is the privileged marker of healthy self-esteem. The trajectory assumed by peer education is that the nascent gay or lesbian person is isolated, and is yet to discover the gay world which will eventually draw them in.

In this study, the men used the peer-education groups as a route out of their social and sexual isolation. In particular they provided an opportunity to meet with men like themselves. The processes of the groups go beyond providing a new circle of friends: they assist men to become gay by transforming their homosexual desire into a gay identity.

As has been recognized in other studies, most of the men we interviewed believed, in retrospect, that they were attracted to boys or men from an early age, well before their knowledge of any gay social networks (Mcintosh, Weeks and Plummer, 1981). David (23) said:

> I have always had a desire to see what other boys had built in their pants, OK. That's something I've always had a desire of.

And Stephen (19) said:

> It was confusing [desiring men], I don't think there was conflict. It was just like, 'What the hell is going on? Is there anybody else [who] feels this?' and stuff. And then there was a special on TV one night about [homosexuality] and I thought well, 'Here we go, that's what I am.'

Our concern is less with the appearance of homosexual desire and the attendant sense of isolation in our subjects than with their recognition of, or entry into a homosexual culture. For some of the men their entry into gay cultural practice was serendipitous. For example, Stephen (21), was accidentally introduced to a homosexual sub-culture at a public toilet or beat: 'I just wanted to actually use the toilet and there was stuff written on the wall and I thought, "Wow! There you go".' The graffiti on the toilet wall directed him to a nearby beach, where he met other men who then introduced him to a local gay social group. Beats thereby provided Stephen with a pathway into gay culture.

Some men have extensive histories of homosexual practice outside notions of gay identity, and make contact with gay culture as a result of their sexual involvement with other men. From around the age of eight, Phillip (26) began having sex with other boys, extending to the playground at school, and then to chance encounters in wider public realms. In his early teens he was picked up on a train and subsequently had anal intercourse for the first time. This man introduced him to the more organized gay culture of Sydney's Oxford Street.

Unlike most of the participants, Phillip was already familiar with homosexual sex, within and outside of gay culture, before he joined the youth group. Other men entered gay culture through different channels, perhaps because they failed to stumble on public and other sex environments, or because personal characteristics resisted their use of such facilities. Robert (19), for example, said: 'You have to have sex with somebody that you know – love more or less.' He equated casual sex, beats and gay venues as places where a physical, non-loving and purely sexual body existed. Robert resisted elements of gay culture he perceived to be outside his desires and values (i.e. beats, gay pubs and clubs). The youth group better facilitated his particular needs, as it was seen as a social rather than a sexual place – as a place where a regular partner might be and indeed was found. Robert therefore was not a *tabula rasa* upon which a gay identity was inscribed. He brought with him an already socially constructed worldview, a part of which included an equation between love and sex. In this sense, gay peer education groups may be seen as expanding the range of possibilities through which men become gay or enter into gay culture.

When Robert (19) disclosed he was gay to his parents he was asked to seek counselling, but he inverted the situation:

> Mum might have said uh, 'Oh, well, we better get you counselling', or whatever, and I said um, I said, 'I don't need counselling, I think you might need counselling', because you know, I knew what I was and um, you have to before you can tell your parents, I think.

Robert encouraged his parents to seek counselling and by his account, 'after different phone calls they got into [a counsellor] with ACON (AIDS Council of NSW)'. 'Ringing around' was enough to put Robert and his parents in contact with an organization waiting for men who are reaching out to explore their homosexuality. ACON helped Robert's parents to accept their son being gay, and Robert's movement toward gayness. He was thus constituted as a gay man in part by participating in a formalized, institutionally mediated, learning process.

Similarly, other interviewees *planned* their coming out. Eugene (25) had been in the army for many years and had a long-term girlfriend. He was aware of his desire for other men but only engaged with those desires in private rumination:

> You had to be 100 per cent formal all the time. But when you'd come home and you'd sit down and have a cup of coffee and you'd think, yea, well such and such wasn't bad looking today, and he was alright and – yea, he wasn't too bad and stuff like that. And that was as far as it would go.

Eugene decided to 'give all that up' (including his female partner), and get assistance in exploring his homosexuality: 'I'm gonna get help . . . I know there's people out there that can help you, it's just a matter of going to the right place.' He made contact with the Gay and Married Men's Association and from there was referred to the peer education youth group at his local AIDS Council.

The men we interviewed typically came to recognize themselves as being homosexual in isolation from other gay people. Their sense of isolation led them to become proactive in searching out a space where their homosexuality could find expression. At this point they were often channelled into pre-existing institutional frameworks through diverse pathways. The youth groups are only one possible point of entry into gay culture and may not be the first. Television and other mass media, for example, were frequently mentioned by the men as elements in their initial recognition of themselves as homosexual and their identification of other homosexual people and places. As such, mass media opened up a possibility of active participation in gay culture and/or homosexual sex. One interviewee's first personal contact within a gay network was through a gay bulletin on the Internet. Others made their first contact through telephone sex lines. Gay youth groups are neither necessary nor sufficient to the development of a gay identity. However, the groups are an emergent site of transition into gayness for young men and may become increasingly important over time.

The Australian Public Health Response to AIDS

The advent of HIV/AIDS has been the catalyst for the formation of a new pathway into gay culture, a pathway which receives institutional and financial support under the umbrella of public health. The recent evaluation of Australia's National HIV/AIDS Strategy notes that 'Peer education and community development have been the key strategies used in the Education and Prevention Program' (Feachem, 1995, p. 108). The precepts of 'the new public health' have guided Australia's response to HIV/AIDS since the mid-1980s. Neal Blewett, Federal Health Minister from 1983 to 1990, summarizes the key strategies as including:

> the involvement of high risk groups in the shaping of public policy; the involvement of patients in decision-making; the respect for the rights of those affected by disease; the justifiable suspicion of the counter-productive consequences of relying on coercion in public health; a recognition of the social dimensions of disease; [and] the mobilisation of affected groups as vital agents for behavioural change. (Blewett, 1993: 24)

This approach was taken by the Australian government not out of an inherent commitment to progressive libertarian views, but because it made good public health sense. Along with much wider tendencies in contemporary 'advanced liberal' government, externally imposed regulation is being increasingly supplanted by self-regulation – and self-regulation extended to ever wider domains of personal conduct (Rose, 1989; Cruikshank, 1993).

HIV emerged in Australia at a time when new public health advocates were beginning to make their voices heard in health bureaucracies (Ballard, 1989). Recognizing that the greatest impact of AIDS would fall on homosexually active men, gay community spokespeople, representing all these men, were included in advisory structures and community-based organizations funded to develop community-action strategies. The success of these policies received empirical endorsement with the research finding from the 1990 Social Aspects of the Prevention of AIDS study which found that 'attachment to an organised gay community and its safe sex education programs is significantly related to successful behaviour change among gay-identified men' (Dowsett, 1990b).

Armed with this finding, gay community HIV-prevention efforts at the beginning of the 1990s embraced peer education as a key strategy. Drawing on earlier models of consciousness-raising, contemporary youth groups use an array of current psychosocial techniques of personal development to help men to become gay. Gay community demands for a community-based response to the impact of the AIDS epidemic thus came to coincide with the public health imperatives to minimize HIV transmission. Added to the haphazard sexual, commercial and social routes of entry to gay cultural practice were systematic, well-advertised government-funded programmes guided by the professional norms of health promotion, counselling and social work. In direct and indirect ways, these new routes to gayness have been crucial to the men in our study.

Peer Education on the Ground

Peer education groups are designed to ensure men at risk of HIV know how to avoid becoming infected. They use two basic methods: imparting information on HIV transmission to change behaviour accordingly, improving self-esteem. ACON's 'Start Making Sense' youth peer education manual states: 'Research clearly shows that self-esteem affects assertiveness and the ability to make safe sex decisions.'

Tim (20) explained why he thought the youth group was called 'Fun and Esteem':

> It's called Fun and Esteem because they do it by, you know, having fun and getting your esteem up, because apparently statistics show that . . . the incidence of AIDS transmission . . . um . . . is very high in people that have been, you know, depressed. And so, yeah, the group's called Fun and Esteem, and if you feel happy with yourself then

maybe, you know, the transmission will drop . . . when I was nineteen
I wasn't having sex or anything . . . I was just playing around with
drugs and stuff like that . . . and that's a pretty abusive thing to do.

Tim's own experience suggests a more complex relationship between self-
esteem and safe sex. He went on to say that he did not like to use condoms
with his new partner: 'I want to be comfortable with him . . . yeah . . . and part
of the comfort, as I said is not using a condom. You see, 'cause I want him . . .
as a relationship.'

Having a relationship was important to Tim and to not use condoms
within a relationship served to define what a relationship was. In part, to use
a condom was, by default, akin to casual sex. The implicit equivalence he
draws between casual sex and condoms may relate to the history of condom
promotion in gay safe sex campaigns, which assumes casual sexual relations
are the norm. For men who value monogamy and who believe themselves to
be in a seroconcordant-negative relationship, the association between condoms
and casual sex may symbolize infidelity and a lack of trust within their relationships. In such contexts condoms may be regarded as intolerable.

Tim had negotiated unprotected anal intercourse with his partner badly.
Although they had told one another they were HIV-negative, there had been
no detailed discussion of sexual history or HIV-testing history. The decision not
to use condoms was made during anal intercourse. Tim's actions would seem
to contradict his own understanding of the rationale of the peer-education
group he attended. Not to use condoms with his regular partner became
intimately bound up with a high self-esteem. As he pointed out, he had had
no sex at the time his self-esteem was lowest. Skilling men to negotiate the
appropriate contexts within which to abandon condoms are crucial topics for
peer education. The example of Tim illustrates that his unsafe sex occurred
precisely when his self-esteem had improved (when he secured a regular
partner) and that this moment was also when he abandoned condoms.

Of the 23 men interviewed in this study, eight reported being in relationships. All eight were not using condoms with their regular partners and
many had poorly negotiated this move. Given these men were moving for
the first time into gay social networks and environments with a high HIV-
prevalence, it is crucial that if they are resisting the use of condoms within
relationships that they develop a capacity to do so in ways that minimize the
risk of HIV-transmission. That is, peer-education groups need to impart sound
negotiated safety principles to their participants.

The Ghettoization of Gayness: Social rather than Individual

Peer-education groups in Australia tend to mark the gay experience as separate from that of straight people. Men enter into peer education with an

already profound sense of difference from their heterosexual peers, but the groups reify that sense of difference into identity. Many of our interviewees were reluctant to identify as gay, either to themselves or to other people. For some of the men, the youth group provided the space to develop a gay iden-tity in a supportive environment. Others initially found the groups incongru-ous to their self-identity. David (19) had recently begun telling his family and straight friends that he was gay but was often reluctant to disclose his gayness to others:

> Maybe 'cause I won't let myself believe either [that I am gay] ... due to my perspective that people know I'm a straight when I'm not ... people see me [as a] trainee, as being straight in certain ways and I don't want to lose that yet ... due to I have my paranoids.

Despite the fear of making a transition, David was in the process of becoming more gay identified and was having to negotiate the negative social con-sequences of such a transition, which, for him, included a loss of social mobility within heterosexual domains.

Paul (19) was also afraid that people would perceive him differently as a gay person and this fear paradoxically moved him away from straight people toward gay people. When he was sixteen he claimed that peer pressure led him to have sex with a girl and that he had to think of a man to get an erection and perform the act. His immersion into gay culture can be read as a retreat from the social demand to be heterosexual. Carl Whitman's 1972 *Gay Manifesto* called San Francisco 'a refugee camp for homosexuals ... we came not because it is so great here, but because it was so bad there' (Whitman, 1972, p. 330). Sydney, too, can be understood as a sanctuary for homosexuality – but it comes at a price, which is to forego heterosexual privilege *and* to adopt a relatively fixed and singular gay identity.

Paul's life is demarcated into exclusively homosexual or heterosexual zones. There was no comfortable transitional area bridging the gap between the two worlds. Class dynamics exacerbated the divide. Paul liked the straight friends from his working-class suburban community better than middle-class inner-city people, whom he associated with dominant gay culture. In the West, he said appreciatively, people are a 'bit wilder'. He spoke of a boss who came from the middle-class eastern suburbs of Sydney who 'sound[ed] gay but was not'. The gay community was understood to be middle-class, and informs his statement that 'my type of person is hard to find' in the inner-city gay scene. As with other interviewees, the western suburbs were under-stood to be masculine and working-class and the inner-city as feminine and middle-class.

Paul felt his peers in the youth group 'spoke a different language'. The predominant social construction of gayness in such groups reproduces some of the exclusions common to dominant gay culture. Despite Paul's resistance to gayness, over the course of a year where he lived and socialized, his identity had become more gay. Albeit brief, his contact with the youth group was a springboard into a wider gay community. Through it Paul came to frequent gay hotels. He could now drive to Oxford Street and visit gay pubs by himself without 'feeling totally paranoid and out of place'.

Tim also had difficulties in moving toward gayness. He dreaded being excluded from broad social participation as a result of desiring men. At the time of the first interview he said: 'I don't want to have to feel as though I'm excluded from anything just because I'm . . . not exclusively heterosexual.' And again: 'I don't want to be part of a gay community, I want to be part of the community, right. I don't want to feel, you know, excluded just because of my sexuality.' A year later Tim remained adamant that gayness was not a criterion for his choice of friends. But over the same period he had moved from an outlying town to Sydney, had developed gay male friends only and lived in an all-gay male household. Despite his avowed preferences, heterosexist social structures and Tim's homosexual desire had moved him consistently toward a gay social life.

Men involved in the youth groups asserted their individuality. Each came to the group with a different mix of homosexual experience and gay sensibility. In order to function effectively, the groups needed to preserve the men's sense that their individuality was being respected and that they were not being turned into clones of one another. They would commonly assert, both on entry to and graduation from the groups, that they were not 'a typical gay man' or really into 'the gay scene'. But despite variations in detail, the men took broadly identical paths. They had been helped to define themselves more comfortably as gay and had moved closer to a defined gay lifestyle. Participation in the youth groups socialized these men into a dominant gay culture. Along with their attitudinal changes, many of the men made life changes which involved moving closer to the epicentre of gay Sydney and heightening their socialization with other gay men.

The Continuing Need for Peer Education

Peer education has been supported as a public health strategy on the basis of the finding that gay community attachment is correlated with better safe sex knowledge by gay men, and increased sexual behaviour change (Kippax *et al.*, 1990). In the five years since that finding was made in 1990, Australian gay men have continued to sustain high levels of safe sexual practice. However, in the intervening five years it has become increasingly evident that inner-city gay Sydney has remained the epicentre of Australia's HIV epidemic.

The Sydney Men and Sexual Health Study (SMASH) is an ongoing longitudinal study of more than 1000 Sydney gay men. Findings from that study indicate that the majority of gay men consistently and successfully employ safe sex strategies. Seventy-six per cent of the men who have some unprotected anal intercourse with their regular partner are in seroconcordant relationships. With more occasional partners, 16 per cent of men sometimes or never used condoms in the previous six months. Interestingly, when looked at over a period of time, it is not the same group of men who are consistently having unsafe sex. That is, a minority of men occasionally do not adhere to safe sex practices. Overwhelmingly, the picture that emerges from the SMASH study is of men who generally practise safe sex. There is no evidence to suggest there is a large group of 'risk-takers' refusing the safe sex message, nor that it is young people or people using particular drugs who are incorrigible unsafe sex practitioners (Prestage *et al.*, 1995; Van de Ven *et al.*, in press).

However, what does emerge from the SMASH study is that gay men are concentrated in inner-city Sydney, and that most men with HIV live in this gay Sydney area. Analysis of the regional distribution of SMASH participants shows: 'respondents living in outer suburban areas were less likely to have been tested for HIV than the respondents living in inner urban areas, or to have tested HIV-positive' (Prestage *et al.*, 1995, p. 32). There were, however, no differences between inner-city and outer-suburban participants in their likelihood to practise safe sex, although outer-suburban participants were less likely to have anal intercourse with occasional partners – a finding that parallels Project SIGMA's findings in relation to London versus other areas in Britain (Davies *et al.*, 1993).

Adding to the picture of a concentration of Australia's HIV epidemic are the findings of a study of recent HIV seroconverters (Kippax *et al.*, 1994). Comparing men who recently seroconverted with a matched control group who remained HIV-negative, there were no differences in relationship status, education, number of casual sexual partners, STDs, drug and alcohol use or attachment to the gay community. The most significant factor associated with seroconversion was living in gay Sydney. In the final analysis, the only other factors found to be significant were receptive anal intercourse as a favourite practice, believing withdrawal to be safe, having an HIV-positive partner and low alcohol consumption.

Conclusions

Since the late 1980s, the Australian policy community has congratulated itself on the effectiveness of the national strategic response to HIV/AIDS and, in particular, the maintenance of a partnership between governments, health professions and the affected communities. The precepts of the new public health are normally credited with providing the policy framework underlying this success. However, the stability of the policy consensus also relies on its conformity with a key 'old public health' value – the containment of disease. Australia's HIV epidemic has remained overwhelmingly confined to gay men and is likely to remain so for the foreseeable future. In this light, the core new public health technique of community development, including assisting homosexually active men to secure their gay identity, also serves the old public health goal of containing the spread of HIV to a community where it is already prevalent.

Peer education is the principal health-education strategy used to skill gay men to operate effectively within gay culture. One of its unintended consequences is to reinforce the divide between heterosexual and homosexual identity and practice. Initial justifications for the public health value of peer education asserted that community attachment and improving self-esteem *per se* reduced HIV risk. In the years since such strategies were first developed, the emphasis has shifted from gay community attachment as a predictor of lower HIV risk to evenly distributed risk practices against a background of the concentration of HIV in the core gay community. We continue to believe that gay community-based peer education is a sound public health response to HIV, but its goals need to be refined.

Peer education is premised on a notion of sameness, reified through the trope of 'coming out' as a manifestation of *authentic being*. In order to give more weight to the diversity of homosexual desire, it is important to make clear the profoundly social nature of homosexuality. Peer-education groups need to realize that they are not only providing a space in which men can be gay, they also provide a space in which to *become* gay or, as Herdt (1992) said, they are a space of 'socialization'.

The sophistication of peer education's understanding of safe and unsafe sex also needs to continue to grow. In fostering a safe sex culture through community development, the various reasons for and contexts of unsafe sex need to be recognized and not reduced to a function of individual personality or self-esteem. For example, data showing that unprotected anal intercourse is common in the context of regular relationships has entailed training and supporting men to have unprotected sex *safely* – that is to say, paying attention to the ways of having and maintaining their HIV-negative seroconcordance.

Above all, peer education must recognize that it channels men into a core gay community and there is a high concentration of HIV within that community. Some current peer education curriculum and practice gives the impression that being properly gay protects against HIV. Positive men tend to participate in peer-support activities with other positive men, but exclude themselves or feel excluded from peer-education activities which become *de facto* HIV-negative peer education. Those positive men who are part of peer-education groups are often reluctant to disclose their status, thus silencing their testimony. That message needs to change. Attaching to gay community today means living with HIV, either directly or in close proximity.

Notes

1 Our use of the term *coming out* assumes a dynamic social process whereby, (1) an individual person recognizes they have an attraction to the same sex, and (2) this attraction is disclosed to other people. The development of a gay identity will differ in relation to individuals and the social context within which they become gay (Davies *et al.*, 1993; Cain, 1991).
2 The interviews were conducted between 1993 and 1995 as a part of the Homosexually Active Men's project at the National Centre in HIV Social Research, Macquarie University, Sydney.

References

BALLARD, J. (1989) 'The politics of AIDS', in H. GARDNER (Ed.) *The Politics of Health: the Australian Experience*, Edinburgh: Churchill Livingstone.

BLEWETT, N. (1993) *AIDS: How We Got Where We Are*, The Keith Harbour Memorial Lecture, Victorian AIDS Council/Gay Men's Health Centre, Melbourne, 26 September 1993.

BRAY, A. (1982) *Homosexuality in Renaissance England*, London: Gay Men's Press.

CAIN, R. (1991) 'Secrecy and disclosure among gay men', *Journal of the History of Sexuality*, **2**, 1, Chicago: The University of Chicago.

CRUIKSHANK, B. (1993) 'Revolutions within: self-government and self-esteem', *Economy and Society*, **22**, p. 3.

DAVIES, P., HICKSON, F., WEATHERBURN, P. and HUNT, A. (1993) *Social Aspects of AIDS: Sex, Gay Men and AIDS*, London: Falmer Press.

DAVIS, T. (1995) 'The diversity of queer politics and the redefinition of sexual identity and community in urban spaces', in D. BELL and G. VALENTINE (Eds) *Mapping Desire*, London, Routledge.

DOWSETT, G. (1990a) 'Reaching Men who have Sex with Men in Australia'. An Overview of AIDS Education: Community Intervention and Community Attachment Strategies, *Australian Journal of Social Issues*, **25**, 3, p. 191.

DOWSETT, G. (1990b) *Summary of Findings from the Social Aspects of the Prevention AIDS Project: Study A*, paper presented at the 3rd National Workshop for Educators of Gay and Bisexual Men, Sydney, October.

FEACHEM, R. (1995) *Valuing the Past . . . Investing in the Future: Evaluation of the National HIV/AIDS Strategy 1993–4 to 1995–6*, Commonwealth Department of Human Health and Services, Canberra: Looking Glass Press.

HERDT, G. (1992) ' "Coming out" as a right of passage: a Chicago study', in G. HERDT (Ed.) *Gay Culture in America: Essays from the Field*, Boston: Beacon Press.

KIPPAX, S., CRAWFORD, J., CONNELL, R., DOWSETT, G., WATSON, L., RODDEN, P., BAXTER, D. *et al.* (1990) *Social Aspects of the Prevention of AIDS Report Number 7: The*

Importance of Gay Community in the Prevention of HIV Transmission, Sydney: Macquarie University.

KIPPAX, S., KALDOR, J., CROFTS, N., HENDRY, O., NOTTS, P., NOBLE, J. (1994) 'Risk Factors for HIV among Homosexually Active Men', paper presented at the 6th Annual Conference of the Australasian Society for HIV Medicine, November.

MCINTOSH, M., WEEKS, J. and PLUMMER, K. (1981) 'Postscript to the homosexual role', in K. PLUMMER (Ed.) *The Making of the Modern Homosexual*, London: Hutchinson.

PRESTAGE, G., KIPPAX, S., CRAWFORD, J., NOBLE, J., BAXTER, D. and COOPER, D. (1995) *Sydney Men and Sexual Health: A Demographic, Behavioural and Clinical Profile of HIV-positive Men in a Sample of Homosexually Active Men in Sydney, Australia*, Macquarie University, Sydney: HIV/AIDS and Society Publications.

ROSE, N. (1989) *Governing the Soul: The Shaping of the Private Self*, London: Routledge.

VAN DE VEN, P., NOBLE, J., KIPPAX, S., PRESTAGE, G., CRAWFORD, J., BAXTER, D. and COOPER, D. (in press) 'Gay youth and their precautionary sexual behaviours: The Sydney Men and Sexual Health Study', *AIDS Education and Prevention*.

WEEKS, J. (1977) *Coming Out: Homosexual Politics in Britain, from the Nineteenth Century to the Present*, London: Quartet Books.

WHITMAN, C. (1972) 'Gay manifesto', in K. JAY and A. YOUNG (Eds) *Out of the Closets*, New York: Jove/Harcourt Brace Jovanovich.

Chapter 14

Sexual Negotiation Strategies of HIV-Positive Gay Men: A Qualitative Approach

Peter Keogh, Susan Beardsell and Sigma Research

Previous studies of HIV-positive gay men have focused either on their contribution to the subsequent spread of the epidemic or the impact of diagnosis and disease progression on psychological wellbeing (Green *et al.*, 1992; Hedge *et al.*, 1992). Studies of sexual behaviour remain rare and findings about the sexual risk behaviour of HIV-positive gay men are largely inconclusive (Higgins *et al.*, 1991; Weatherburn *et al.*, 1993). However, differences in psychosexual adjustment have been found between samples of HIV-positive gay men and their HIV-negative counterparts. For instance, high levels of sexual dysfunction such as erectile failure and psychosexual morbidity such as loss of sexual pleasure, have been found both in samples of HIV-positive men (Brown and Pace, 1989; Jones, Klimes and Catalan, 1994) and in comparative studies of HIV-positive and HIV-negative gay men (Meyer-Bahlburg *et al.*, 1991). However, many studies of the effects of HIV on sexual behaviour deliberately study only respondents who have been living with HIV for a number of years (Jones, Klimes and Catalan, 1994) and avoid any considerations of adjustment effects to a new diagnosis by concentrating on long-term sexual behaviour patterns. Other studies concentrate on men with symptomatic HIV disease in order to investigate the effects of various drugs on sexual functioning and physiological impairment (Tindall, Forde and Cooper, 1992).

The period following an HIV diagnosis is largely ignored by many researchers precisely because the unpredictable reactions shown by newly diagnosed people do not easily lend themselves to measurement or interpretation. However, these initial effects are of central importance to understanding the later development of successful coping strategies. Moreover, there is little or no research into HIV-positive gay men's experiences of sex and the motivations behind their sexual decision-making. Yet higher levels of sexual dysfunction and of psychosexual morbidity suggest that the experience of sex and sexual negotiation may differ between HIV-positive and HIV-negative or untested men. Information on these differences is vital to understanding quantitative studies of sexual behaviour and important in the formulation of sexual health campaigns for HIV-positive gay men.

This chapter details some of the results of a qualitative study which investigated the experience of sex and sexual negotiation of HIV-positive gay men living in London.[1] The research focuses first on the immediate impact of an HIV diagnosis on sex and sexual negotiation and, second, on attitudes towards the subject of reinfection with HIV and cross-infection with other STDs. Finally, we outline the implications of this research for sexual health promotion with members of this group.

The aim of this study was to gain a detailed understanding of the experience of sex and sexual negotiation of HIV-positive men. To do this, ten focused discussion groups were convened. The groups were facilitated by a senior researcher and observed by a second researcher who examined the group dynamics and levels of concurrence among group members (Basch, 1987; Krueger, 1988). Internal reliability was ensured by using a third researcher to conduct content analysis independently (Kirk and Miller, 1986; Henwood and Pidgeon, 1992). The groups were tape-recorded and full transcripts were made. Grounded theory methods were used (Glaser and Strauss, 1967; Rennie, Phillips and Quartaro, 1988; Henwood and Pidgeon, 1992) to analyse the data. In the first four groups, participants were asked to discuss the effects of an HIV diagnosis on their social and sexual lives, particularly in the six months following diagnosis. Participants were encouraged to give examples of critical incidents and these examples were discussed by the group. An initial analysis was carried out on the resulting transcripts from which key themes emerged. In the following three groups, these themes were used to inform and amend questioning routes. The final three groups focused on the results of the previous seven. Transcripts of all ten groups were subjected to a secondary thematic content analysis. Respondents were recruited through advertisements in the London gay press, at gay pubs and clubs and at AIDS Service Organizations. The groups took place in London over seven months in 1994.

Sample

Ninety men participated in ten groups. The mean age of the sample was 31 years (range 21–54). Seventy-eight men were white European, eight were white non-European. Two men were African–Caribbean, one was African and one was Asian. The mean number of years since an HIV diagnosis was two-and-a-half with a range from three months to nine years. Eight men had an AIDS diagnosis.

Sexual Response to a Positive HIV Diagnosis

Respondents characterized their immediate response to an HIV diagnosis in terms of either an increase or decrease in numbers of sexual partners. The exceptions were men already in long-term or monogamous relationships who tended to stay the same. Responses to diagnosis could be arranged along a distinct continuum, the polar points of which are giving up sexual contact for a period (celibacy) and increasing the number of 'casual' or anonymous sexual partners (sexual anonymity). Most of the men had experienced one or the other of these two reactions to a lesser or greater degree. Moreover, respondents easily recognized them as a common reaction among their peers.

Respondents characterized these reactions as emerging from a new and unpredicted anxiety about their perceived inability to negotiate sex now that they had a different HIV status. Two strong themes emerged relating to this anxiety. The first was a concern about disclosing their HIV status to a sexual partner. The second was a concern about being solely responsible for the safety of a sexual encounter – that is, concerns about infecting sexual partners.

Disclosure

Difficulties in disclosing HIV status to potential partners often arose. Respondents experienced their partners' reactions as problematic. First, they feared sexual rejection. Many had experienced this rejection, although the necessity to anticipate it was perceived as more damaging than actual rejection.

> and then, after all that chatting up and effort, having to anticipate the worst automatically, that this one might just be the one who will throw a real wobbly . . . to prepare yourself for that every time you have sex. I used to really enjoy cruising, you know, the chase, but this just wears you down.

Thus approaching a prospective partner for sex had become a difficult and unpleasant experience. Even when potential partners responded positively to a disclosure, this response was not always appropriate and could lead to an inordinate interest from sexual partners in the respondent's HIV disease. Respondents reported having to field enquiries about their general state of health, whether their friends had died, etc. in an encounter which was supposed to be enjoyable and sexual. 'You spend the whole evening talking about being sick and people dying. They don't seem to want to know anything about you, just your HIV. It's really rather depressing, like you're a freak or something.' Respondents experienced this as an invasion of privacy or as simply distressing. They therefore feel a substantial disincentive to disclose.

Responsibility

If respondents did not disclose their HIV status to sexual partners, they felt that *they* had to take complete responsibility for the safety of the sexual encounter. The greatest fear in this context was accidentally infecting a partner, either through a faulty or broken condom or through oral sex. Men were particularly worried about ejaculating in the mouth of their partners or the infectivity of their pre-ejaculate. 'What if the condom breaks and you don't notice? What do you tell him after if you haven't told him you're HIV already? There's no way to tell him then.'

Respondents also worried about the effects of alcohol or drugs on their own or their partners' judgement. They also feared recriminations from sexual partners who might subsequently find out that they were HIV-positive, even if the encounter was safe. In limited social networks of gay men, this possibility is very real:

> My history is that a lot of people I sleep with are friends of friends. They're people I know. I mean a lot of my gay friends have become friends of mine usually after we've had sex and so that if I don't tell them and they discover from somebody else, then, you know, that becomes a barrier, so I need to tell people, but I'm scared.

Finally, respondents were worried in case a casual sexual encounter resulted in a friendship or relationship, which many desired, but which would be jeopardized when they subsequently disclosed their status. This feeling of responsibility and secrecy was experienced by many as a barrier to intimacy and made sexual encounters stressful:

> I'd like to think that I'll fall in love again, and you think, now, where does that happen? It happens between the sheets or over breakfast when you realize 'I really like him.' I won't let myself feel that because I know that as soon as I tell him, he'll run a mile.

Respondents reported being in a double bind. If they disclosed their HIV status, they risked negative or inappropriate reactions which made sexual encounters problematic. If they did not disclose, they risked being found out or having to disclose after they had perhaps risked infecting a partner. Dealing with these concerns shortly after the shock of a positive HIV-diagnosis made sexual negotiation difficult.

The key to these problems was their concern with sexual *negotiation* as opposed to sex itself. Consequently, an immediate coping reaction was to obviate the need for negotiation in a sexual encounter. Respondents who did not stop sex after a diagnosis reported a preference for having no emotional or social connection with their partners. For some, this meant a casual encounter; others reported 'not wanting to see the face' of their partners. These men did not desire to have unprotected sex with their partners, they merely did not want to have to verbally negotiate the sexual encounter.

Thus the seemingly opposed reactions – celibacy and sexual anonymity – are different responses to the same problem: that is, a new and increased complexity in sexual negotiation. Men cope with this difficulty by either ceasing to have sex or having anonymous or 'casual sex' for which little or no verbal negotiation is necessary.

Other Coping Strategies

Although most respondents had experienced these immediate reactions to a diagnosis, many had subsequently moved on to more successful sexual negotiation. There were four main strategies in achieving this. First, respondents found that they had to re-learn the negotiation of sex. Many talked about acquiring new skills which they equated with learning how to 'cruise' and 'pick up' when they first became sexually active. They also learned who to tell:

P1: Well, you just sit there and listen to them for a while, you generally know whether or not to tell them.

P2: How do you judge that?

P1: Well, if they're older for one, that helps, or if they haven't come out with anything that says, you know, 'I'm scared of AIDS' or if they talk about friends who have it. A good way is to bring AIDS into the conversation and see how they react, that's always a good one.

And they learned when was the best time to tell:

I always have to know them first and I always have to go to either my place or their place. It's not always that I decide to tell them and now, I suppose, because of the length of time [since diagnosis]. I mean in your case (to P2) it's a short period. I do get to know whether to tell them in the place I meet them or I gauge whether to tell them when I get home; and with some people, I wait until we are going to start because you have to judge what some people want and you do get a reaction sometimes.

Men felt that these strategies were informed by self-confidence and a kind of 'sixth sense':

> Well, you've just got to get yourself into the right frame of mind, you've got to decide to be upfront and not think too much about the consequences.

> It's like cruising, you gradually get a sense for it, when the right time is to dive in with the information.

Prolonged contact with either formal or informal support networks of other HIV-positive gay men was seen as vital to the acquisition of these skills about sex and sexual negotiation. The advice and support gained from these networks was also useful in the development of further sexual health strategies. One of these was learning how to deal positively with rejection. Men learned to realize that sexual rejection was not a rejection of themselves, rather it was a rejection of HIV. However, ongoing support was seen as essential to maintaining this strategy. Peer support was also necessary in the development of a further strategy. This was to off-load the overwhelming sense of responsibility for the sexual safety of the encounter. By realizing that their partner was equally but differently responsible within the sexual encounter, men could begin to be more relaxed about sex. However, they still needed peer support to deal with mishaps such as a condom breaking. Thus the acquisition of these skills made it possible for respondents to make choices about disclosure with greater confidence without feeling solely responsible for any adverse consequences of the encounter.

Finally, many men expressed a preference for other HIV-positive sexual partners, for a variety of reasons. It reduced the difficulties associated with negotiating sex with an HIV-negative partner: 'You find that you're both positive, well, there's nothing more to be said, you just go off and clinch the deal.' Men also felt a certain emotional closeness and empathy with HIV-positive partners which they did not necessarily feel with men who did not know their own status:

> I always find that I want to speak to him that much more to see what he thinks of HIV. There's nothing worse than someone saying something really stupid in the middle of sex, or having cold feet because this is the first time they've done it with someone who has it. I don't mind if that happens, but I like to know what I'm in for.

> if he's positive as well, you always talk about this drug and that and, you know, 'where do you go and who do you know', but there's more and that is that you're on the same planet as him.

And the resulting sex was felt to be more satisfying since they felt more at ease in the sexual encounter.

> no matter what, you know that you can't infect him, you just know
> it for sure.

> If the condom slips, it's not the end of the world, you're not going
> to have a gibbering wreck on your hands.

Some men also concluded that they could have unprotected anal intercourse
without any adverse health consequences.

Analysis of comments on the development of longer-term strategies
towards sexual negotiation revealed a general dissatisfaction with the sexual
health advice from medical and mental health professionals.

> The health adviser at the clinic said you don't have to tell anybody
> about your status. Mutual responsibility as long as you're careful.
> That's the most useless advice I've ever had.

There were three reasons for this dissatisfaction. First, the advice failed to
recognize the fact that gay men often live within small community networks
where both sexual and social interactions coalesce. Second, it did not recognize the central role that specifically sexual interaction plays in the lives of
many gay men; and finally, gay men were unused to taking advice on sexual
matters from medical sources.

Respondents found prolonged interpersonal contact with other HIV-
positive gay men most useful. It was clear that formal and informal support
networks were vital for the development of skills and as a source of support.
For some, they also served as a source of HIV-positive sexual partners.

Re-infection and Cross-infection with HIV and Other STDs

Large cohort studies of gay men's sexual behaviour have shown that a positive HIV diagnosis does not stop gay men engaging in unprotected anal intercourse (UAI) (Van Griensven *et al*, 1989; Davies *et al*, 1993; Weatherburn *et
al*, 1993). Hickson *et al* (1994) identified some of the circumstances in which
gay men engage in UAI as being when they know or assume that their partners
HIV status is the same as their own. Most importantly this study showed that
for most men, UAI was a matter of personal choice and was rarely accidental
or not premeditated.

Many of the respondents had engaged in UAI since their diagnosis and
all had been asked by partners to do so. Therefore, although the practice of
UAI may not be the norm, all the men were aware that it occurs and had considered engaging in it. The implications of this are great, as respondents were
reporting making choices about UAI without the support of health-promotion

campaigns. We were prompted therefore to examine the discourse around re-infection and cross-infection. Attitudes of respondents towards the issue fell into four categories. Some saw re- and cross-infection as a theoretical possibility which had been mentioned only in medical terms. 'Yes, I've read about different strains of the virus, but it all seems so ridiculous. No one's ever explained how one differs to another.' Others felt that if their partner was from the same place and had had a similar sexual history, he would probably come from the same pool of infection. 'Aren't other strains from different countries? . . . I generally only have sex with gay men from London and, surely, we all have the same thing.'

Some men felt that they had been warned about this form of infection from their doctors, but were not used to taking medical advice on sexual matters.

> My doctor told me and P. about it but, to be honest, I never listen to anything that anybody has to say about sex in that clinic. They've never given me any reason to suspect that they are any authority on that subject.

Finally, others had the attitude that now they had contracted HIV, they had got 'the big one' and did not see why they should now be worried about other STDs. 'Look, compared to HIV, a dose of the clap is nothing.'

What is significant is not only the level of ignorance about re-infection, other strains of HIV and the health risks of contracting other STDs but also the extent to which information, though received, was ignored. We explored these attitudes further and identified two themes. First, when respondents referred to advice they had been given on this subject they said that it had always originated from a medical source. Second, any discussion on this subject was always accompanied by discussions about anal intercourse. These two themes are explained in more detail.

Advice from Medical Sources

When the facilitator prompted the group on re- and cross-infection, the resulting discussion was always accompanied by comments about medical advice. Men talked about this issue in relation to having read about it in a medical journal or having been told about it by their doctor or other medical practitioner. Some mentioned that they mistrusted the advice of doctors on medical matters. Others said that because they had not seen the issue mentioned within gay media or by gay community sources, they had the impression that the risk was not particularly great. Research has shown how gay men rely heavily on gay community sources and the gay media for their information on sexual matters (Keogh *et al.*, 1994). It is likely, therefore, that many gay men are not taking this issue seriously enough simply because they do not see it covered in the gay press, in leaflets or on posters.

Anal Intercourse

The issue also arose when the men discussed anal intercourse and the decision of whether or not to use a condom. Re-infection and infection with other STDs was always used as a reason for not engaging in UAI. Whereas discussion of the dangers of contracting other STDs through UAI was common, there was not a single mention of the dangers of oral transmission of STDs. Therefore, although many STDs can be transmitted both orally and anally, the men only recognized UAI as a pertinent risk behaviour in this context. This conflation of the dangers of STDs with UAI had the effect of shifting attention away from STDs and on to the much more contentious issue of whether or not to use a condom. Men seemed to use re- and cross-infection as reasons not to engage in UAI rather then thinking of them as distinct health issues. Simply put, the issue of re- and cross-infection and STDs appears to have been subsumed within a much more contentious debate (UAI), thus diminishing its significance.

Discussion

In this study we have explained changes in sexual functioning in some detail. The use of qualitative methods have been extremely useful in studying an area the complexity of which does not easily yield to quantitative measurement. By concentrating on detailed accounts of sexual encounters and accompanying reactions and emotions, we have shown how a diagnosis can have an impact on sexual functioning in a way that has little to do with physiological or sexual dysfunction or individual psychosexual pathology. Rather, we have identified short-term reactions to an extremely complex sexual situation.

Decreases in sexual activity or celibacy both in HIV-positive individuals generally (Green, 1993) and specifically in HIV-positive gay men (Kaplan, Spira and Fishbain, 1988) have been documented. However, accounts of increases in numbers sexual partners are rare, and those that exist have been interpreted as 'denial' of a diagnosis (Green, 1993). We conclude, however, that many gay men who increase the numbers of their sexual partners do so precisely because they are intensely aware of their recent diagnosis. Their use of 'casual' or anonymous sexual partners obviates the need to discuss their status with sexual partners and allows them to continue to have sex.

What is significant about the two reactions we have identified (celibacy and sexual anonymity) is that they are relational: that is, dependent on the perceived, predicted and actual attitudes of sexual partners. They are not indicative of individual pathology, nor did they seem to be related to low self esteem, embarrassment or feeling sexually unattractive.

The short-term strategies we have identified are transitory and mark a phase in the adjustment to an HIV diagnosis. Men later appeared to move to adopt longer-term strategies which included assessing partners' attitudes and coping with rejection and sexual responsibility. In order to develop these strategies, men relied on informal and formal support networks of other HIV-positive gay men. Men did not rely on institutional advice, such as that from medical personnel, sexual health advisers or mental health professionals. Therefore, we conclude that peer support and advice is vital for HIV-positive gay men to develop appropriate coping strategies, at least towards sexual negotiation.

Men did not seem to take the issues of re- and cross-infection and infection with other STDs very seriously. This is because they have not been identified as distinct health issues outside medical contexts and distinct from the far more contentious context of UAI. Thus appropriate information is needed on these issues which should be disseminated through community media and peer networks.

In conclusion, this study identified two main challenges for health promotion with HIV-positive gay men. The first is to provide sexual health promotion which does not simplify nor provide singular solutions to problems such as the negotiation of sexual encounters as an HIV-positive gay man. The second is to provide complex information on sexual health issues (such as re- and cross-infection) in ways that are culturally appropriate to gay men. Sexual health promotion with this constituency could operate following two broad strategies.

The first is experiential/skills-based learning. The men emphasized how the negotiation of a healthy sex life for HIV-positive gay men was dependent on the acquisition of skills. For many, these skills had been gained through interaction with other HIV-positive gay men. Therefore, experiental workshops with an emphasis on the development of skills and empowerment in relation to healthy sex would seem appropriate. These workshops could cover a number of areas such as disclosure and non-disclosure; responsibility for safety; sex with partners of the same HIV status/different status; and unprotected anal intercourse.

The second strategy might involve print and literature campaigns. These campaigns could seek to inform this constituency on a range of subjects which might include HIV testing, including information on the implications of a positive HIV test result on sex, testing within partnerships and the implications of having both concordant and discordant test results; advice on how to cope with a positive diagnosis, aiming to reassure and suggest ways in which solutions can be formulated rather than giving simple solutions to problems; advice on sex with partners of the same and different HIV status; advice on the options open to HIV men about unprotected anal intercourse; and advice on cross- and re-infection, covering a range of harmful diseases that can be transmitted sexually.

Note

1   This research had two sources of funding: first, joint funding by Camden and Islington Community Health Services NHS Trust Health Promotion Service and the London Borough of Camden; second, the Terrence Higgins Trust.

References

BASCH, E. (1987) 'Focus group interview: an underutilised research technique for improving theory and practice in health education', *Health Education Quarterly*, **14**, 4, pp. 411–48.

BROWN, G. and PACE, J. (1989) 'Reduced sexual activity in HIV infected homosexual men', *Journal of the American Medical Association*, **261**, p. 2503.

DAVIES, P., HICKSON, F.C.I., WEATHERBURN, P. and HUNT, A. (1993) *Sex, Gay men and AIDS*, London, Falmer Press.

GLASER, B.G. and STRAUSS, A.L. (1967) *Discovery of Grounded Theory: Strategies for Qualitative Research*, Chicago: AVC.

GREEN, G. (1993) *Positive Sex: The Sexual Relationships of a Cohort of Men and Woman Following an HIV-positive Diagnosis*, oral presentation given at VII Conference on Social Aspects of AIDS, 3 July, London: South Bank University.

GREEN, J., HENDERSON, F., TYRER, P. and HEDGE, B. (1992) *Subjective Quality of Life in Persons with HIV Disease*, poster presentation for VIII International Conference on AIDS, 19–24 July, Amsterdam, PO-B-3565.

HEDGE, B., SLAUGHTER, J., FLYNN, R. and GREEN, J. (1992) *Coping with HIV Disease: Successful Attributes and Strategies*, poster presentation for VIII International Conference on AIDS, 19–24 July, Amsterdam, PO-B-1691.

HENWOOD, J.L. and PIDGEON, N.F. (1992) 'Qualitative research and psychological theorizing', *British Journal of Psychology*, **83**, pp. 97–111.

HICKSON, F.C.I., WEATHERBURN, P., KEOGH, P. and DAVIES, P. (1994) *Perceptions of Partners' Status and Unprotected Anal Intercourse (UAI) among Gay Men*, oral presentation for the 2nd International Conference on Biopsychosocial Aspects of HIV Infection, Brighton, UK, 7–10 July, W4.2.

HIGGINS, D.L., GALAVOTTI, C., O'REILLY, K.R. *et al.* (1991) 'Evidence for the effects of HIV antibody counselling and testing on risk behaviours', *Journal of the American Medical Association*, **226**, pp. 2419–29.

JONES, M., KLIMES, I. and CATALAN, J. (1994) 'Psychosexual problems in people with HIV infection: controlled study of gay men and men with haemophilia', *AIDS Care*, **6**, 5, pp. 587–93.

KAPLAN, J., SPIRA, T. and FISHBAIN, D. (1988) 'Reasons for decrease in sexual activity amongst homosexual men with HIV infection', *Journal of the American Medical Association*, **260**, pp. 2836–7.

KEOGH, P., WEATHERBURN, P., DAVIES, P. and Hickson, F.C.I. (1994) *A Comparitive Evaluation of Three Different HIV Prevention Print Campaigns Aimed at Gay and Bisexual Men in the UK*, oral presentation for the 2nd International Conference on Biopsychosocial Aspects of HIV Infection, Brighton, UK, 7–10 July, IP5.4.

KIRK, J. and MILLER, M.L. (1986) 'Reliability and validity in qualitative research', *Sage University Series on Qualitative Research Methods (Vol 1)*, Beverly Hills, CA: Sage.

KRUEGER, R. (1988) *Focus Groups: a Practical Guide for Applied Research*, Newbury Park, CA: Sage.

MEYER-MAHLBURG, H., EXNER, T. and LORENZ, G., *et al.* (1991) 'Sexual risk behaviour, sexual functioning and HIV disease progression in gay men', *Journal of Sex Research*, **28**, pp. 3–27.

RENNIE, D., PHILLIPS, J. and QUARTARO, G. (1988) 'Grounded theory: a promising approach to conceptualization in psychology?', *Canadian Psychology/Psychologie Canadienne*, **29**, 2, pp. 139–51.

TINDALL, B., FORDE, S. and COOPER, D.A. (1992) *Self-reported Sexual Dysfunction in Advanced HIV Disease*, poster presentation for VIII International Conference on AIDS, 19–24 July, Amsterdam, PO-B-3564.

VAN GRIENSVEN, J.P.G., DE VROOM, E.M.M., GOUDSMIDT, J. and COUTHINO, R.A. (1989) 'Changes in sexual behaviour and the fall in incidence if HIV infection among homosexual men', *British Medical Journal*, **298**, pp. 218–21.

WEATHERBURN, P., DAVIES, P.M., HICKSON, F.C.I., COXON, A.P.M. and MACMANUS, T.J. (1993) *Sexual Behaviour among HIV Antibody Positive Gay Men*, poster presentation for IX International Conference on AIDS, 6–11 June, Berlin, PO-D20-3999.

Notes on Contributors

Derek Adam-Smith is co-director of the Centre for AIDS and Employment Research at Portsmouth Business School. He has researched and written widely on the employment implications of HIV/AIDS and with David Goss is author of *Organizing AIDS: Workplace and Organizational Responses to the HIV/AIDS Epidemic*, Taylor & Francis, 1995.

Peter Aggleton is Professor in Education, Director of the Thomas Coram Research Unit and Associate Director of the Health and Education Research Unit at the Institute of Education, University of London. He has worked internationally in HIV/AIDS health promotion for more than ten years and was chief of Social and Behavioural Studies and Support within the World Health Organization's Global Programme on AIDS between 1992 and 1994. He provides technical support to a range of research projects in developing countries for UNAIDS. His most recent publication is *Bisexualities and AIDS: International Perspectives*, Taylor & Francis, 1996.

Anthony Bainbridge is employed as a Psychological Development Officer by Stockton Social Services. He is currently studying for a PhD at Lancaster University in the area of HIV/AIDS research.

Maura Banim is senior lecturer in social policy at the University of Sunderland. She has carried out research in the area of sexual health, especially in relation to young people, peer education and HIV/AIDS. She is currently working on a project funded by the Northern and Yorkshire Regional Health Authority addressing the sexual health needs of disabled people in Cleveland. This aims to involve disabled people in the development of relevant and appropriate sexual health promotion.

Michael Bartos is a research fellow in the National Centre in HIV Social Research at Macquarie University, Sydney, Australia, working on gay men, sexuality and AIDS. His doctoral research at La Trobe University is concerned with the government of sexuality in Australia, as it has been reorganized by

HIV/AIDS. He has had extensive involvement with community-based AIDS organizations, and was for two years President of the Victorian AIDS Council/Gay Men's Health Centre.

Nigel Beail is a consultant clinical psychologist at Barnsley Community and Priority Services NHS Trust and lecturer in clinical psychology at the University of Sheffield. His current research concerns the process and outcome of psychodynamic psychotherapy with people with intellectual disabilities.

Sue Beardsell is a senior research fellow with Sigma Research based in Brixton, London, and affiliated with the University of Portsmouth. Her most recent major research projects include a two-year qualitative study of psychosocial issues in HIV testing, for the Department of Health, and a Review of GUM Services in Central London for the Inner London HIV Health Commissioners' Group.

Luan Bruce is currently a needle-exchange worker with Drugs Action, a voluntary drugs agency providing information, advice and support to drug users, their families and friends in the Aberdeen area. Before taking up this post, she was employed as research assistant on a study of HIV prevalence among injecting drug users.

Sharon Cahill is currently undertaking a PhD on 'Women's experience of anger: social and personal perspectives' at Glasgow Caledonian University. She has also researched in the area of sexual health, disability and evaluating health education and promotion.

June Crawford is a research consultant to the National Centre in HIV Social Research at Macquarie University, Australia, where she has been involved in HIV/AIDS research since 1987. Her background is in social psychology and research methodology. She currently divides her research interests between the Sydney Men and Sexual Health (SMASH) cohort study and a project documenting the experiences of women living with HIV. Recent publications have appeared in *Feminism and Psychology* and *Venereology*.

Colm Crowley lectures in psychology and counselling at the Institute of Education, University of London. His involvement in the HIV/AIDS voluntary sector has included Frontliners' training team and running a hospital-based support group for partners and affected family members. His publications include, with Susan Hallam, a psychological study of partners and family members living with HIV and AIDS in *AIDS in Europe – The Behavioural Aspect, Vol. 5: Cure and Care*, Edition Sigma, 1995; and, with Rayah Feldman, *HIV Services in a London Borough*, South Bank University, in press.

Peter Davies is Professor in the Sociology of Health and Director of Research in the School of Health Studies at the University of Portsmouth. He is a

Director of SIGMA Research and author of *Key Texts in Multidimensional Scaling*, Heinemann, 1982; *Images of Social Stratification*, Sage, 1985; and co-author, with Ford Hickson, Peter Weatherburn and Andrew Hunt, of *Sex, Gay Men and AIDS*, Taylor & Francis, 1993. He is editor, with Peter Aggleton and Graham Hart, of *AIDS: Responses, Interventions and Care*, Taylor & Francis, 1991; *AIDS: Risk, Rights and Reason*, Taylor & Francis, 1992; *AIDS: Facing the Second Decade*, Taylor & Francis, 1993; *AIDS: Foundations for the Future*, Taylor & Francis, 1994 and *AIDS: Safety, Sexuality and Risk*, Taylor & Francis, 1995.

Katie Deverell is a researcher who has worked in the field related to HIV-prevention since 1988. Much of her research has been concerned with gay and bisexual men and has focused on evaluation and service development. She is currently completing a PhD which focuses on how HIV-prevention outreach workers construct boundaries at work. Her publications include, with Alan Prout, *Working with Diversity: Building Communities Evaluating the MESMAC Project*, London, Health Education Authority, 1995.

Mark Edwards is a lecturer in the Foreign Affairs and Trade Program at the Canberra campus of Monash University. He has taught in the fields of Australian public policy and Australian politics. He is currently completing his PhD, which analyses the use of health promotion as a policy tool in Australia and its relevance to the Australian response to HIV/AIDS.

Rayah Feldman is principal lecturer in primary and community health research at South Bank University, London. She has been involved in research on HIV/AIDS since 1991, especially in relation to social care, and is currently engaged in evaluating the impact of the East London Childcare Initiative. She has also published work on women's health and on development issues in Africa, with special reference to women.

Paul Flowers is a sexual health research fellow at the MRC Medical Sociology Unit, University of Glasgow. He is currently involved in the design and evaluation of an intervention targeting gay men and their HIV-risk related behaviours.

Fiona Goss is a research assistant in the Business School at the University of Portsmouth, currently researching disability and employment.

Alison Guy is a senior lecturer in psychology at the University of Teesside. She formerly worked as an AIDS educator in South Tyneside. She has carried out research in the area of sexual health, especially in relation to young people, peer education and HIV/AIDS, since 1989. She is currently working on a project funded by the Northern and Yorkshire Regional Health Authority addressing the sexual health needs of disabled people in Cleveland. This aims to involve disabled people in the development of relevant and appropriate sexual health promotion.

Graham Hart is assistant director of the MRC Medical Sociology Unit, University of Glasgow, where he directs a programme of research on sexual and reproductive health. He has undertaken studies of risk in gay men, injecting drug users and sex workers, and published widely in the HIV/AIDS field. He is co-editor of the journal *AIDS Care*, and general editor of the forthcoming series of books *Health, Risk and Society*, UCL Press.

Roger Ingham is reader in health and community psychology at the University of Southampton, where he is also director of the Centre for Sexual Health Research. His interests in sexual health started almost ten years ago when he received an ESRC grant to explore contextual aspects of heterosexual conduct. Since then he has been involved in a range of projects, including work for the World Health Organization, the Health Education Authority and the Department of Health. He has recently coordinated a European Commission Concerted Action which involved developing a qualitative research protocol for use in different countries to enable the collection of comparative material on heterosexual conduct.

Emily Jaramazović was a research associate on the study of sexual health alliances described in this book, followed by two years working on an EC-funded Concerted Action, coordinated by Roger Ingham, developing a protocol for use in different countries. This involved extensive fieldwork through detailed interviews and focus group discussions with young people in Britain and The Netherlands; pilot work was conducted in ten further European countries.

Peter Keogh is a senior research fellow with Sigma Research, based in Brixton, London, and affiliated with the University of Portsmouth. In addition to this work on HIV-positive gay men and a range of pre-testing and evaluation projects, he has spent much of the last two years working on a multisite research and development project on Public Sex Environments and Safer Sex, for the former North Thames Regional Health Authority.

Susan Kippax is director of the National Centre in HIV Social Research at Macquarie University, Australia. She has been involved in many aspects of HIV/AIDS research since 1986, and is the author of numerous publications on the social aspects of AIDS. Her publications have appeared in a number of journals, and (with R.W. Connell, C.W. Dowsett and J. Crawford) she is co-author of *Sustaining Safe Sex: Gay Communities Respond to AIDS*, Taylor & Francis, 1993.

Sonia Lawless has been a researcher on the Women Living with HIV and AIDS project at the National Centre in HIV Social Research, Macquarie University, Australia. She is a committed advocate for HIV-positive women.

Krista Maxwell is a research associate in the Department of Public Health Medicine, United Medical and Dental Schools (UMDS), St Thomas' Hospital. She is currently working on an anthropological study of pain in sickle cell disease.

Anne-Lise Middelthon is a researcher in the Section for Medical Anthropology, Institute for Community Medicine, University of Oslo. She is currently working on a research project on young gay men and their coping strategies towards the HIV epidemic. She has worked on different aspects of the HIV epidemic since 1985, including eight years in the Norwegian AIDS Programme.

Kate Philip is a research fellow in the Department of Education, University of Aberdeen. She has been involved in a number of studies on health, young people and drug use and (with L.B. Hendry and J. Shucksmith) is co-author of *Educating for Health, School and Community Approaches with Adolescents*, Cassell, 1995. She is currently involved in a study exploring the role of mentoring in young people's lives and a review of services for women drug users in Scotland.

Paschal Sheeran is a lecturer in social psychology at the University of Sheffield. His research mainly concerns the self-regulation of behaviour. This has involved applications of motivational and volitional accounts of action to health-risk and HIV-preventive behaviours. He also researches the social psychology of identity, especially the impact of culture and social structural position on self-conception.

Janet Shucksmith is senior lecturer in the Department of Education, University of Aberdeen. She has recently completed a study of young people's perceptions of their own health needs. She has co-authored a number of books including *Young People, Leisure and Lifestyles*, Routledge, 1993, and has undertaken a range of research studies on young people and health. She is currently involved in a locality study of community needs in relation to drug misuse and a review of services for women drug users in Scotland.

Neil Small is senior research fellow at the University of Sheffield and the Trent Palliative Care Centre. His research interests currently centre on the care of dying people. He is the author of *Politics and Planning in the NHS*, Open University Press, 1989, and *AIDS, the Challenge: Understanding, Education and Care*, Avebury, 1993.

Gary Smith is a research officer at the National Centre in HIV Social Research, Macquarie University, Sydney, Australia. He began a PhD thesis at Macquarie University in 1996 and is concerned with the representations and practices of anal eroticism in the pre- and post-AIDS era.

Jonathan A. Smith is a lecturer in psychology at the University of Sheffield. He conducts research on self and identity, life transitions and the psychology of health and illness. He is also interested in debates around qualitative approaches in psychology.

Diane Stevens graduated in psychology from the University of Southampton. Her doctoral work involved exploring the contextual aspects of sexual conduct in young people, including looking at the interpretation of terminology, mutual (mis)understandings between parents and their children, and a discursive analysis of the 1992 House of Lords debates on sex education in schools. She worked for one year on the EC funded Concerted Action, coordinated by Roger Ingham, and is currently teaching psychology at a higher education college in Southampton.

Index